Water
The Ultimate Cure

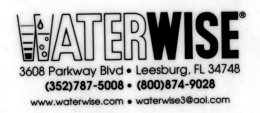

WATERWISE®
3608 Parkway Blvd • Leesburg, FL 34748
(352)787-5008 • (800)874-9028
www.waterwise.com • waterwise3@aol.com

Water
The Ultimate Cure

**Discover Why Water Is the Most
Important Ingredient in Your Diet and
Find Out Which Water is Right for You**

Introduction by
Dr. F. Batmanghelidj, MD

by Steve Meyerowitz

Distributed by
Book Publishing Company
PO Box 99, Summertown, TN 38483
888-260-8458. 931-964-3571. Fax 931-964-3518

Printed in the United States of America
ISBN 1-878736-20-5, Paperback

Library of Congress Control Number: 2001119107

Cover design by Meredith Morford, www.Planet-color.com

Disclaimer: The information in this book is for educational
purposes only. It is not medical advice, nor is it intended to
replace the advice of your physician. Consult a licensed health
professional for diagnosis and treatment of illness and injuries,
for advice regarding medications, and before making changes to
your diet or exercise program.

Distributed by
Book Publishing Company
PO Box 99, Summertown, TN 38483
888-260-8458. 931-964-3571. Fax 931-964-3518
http://bookpubco.com   e-mail: bookpubl@usit.net

Table of Contents

Don't Treat Thirst with Medications
by Dr. F. Batmanghelidj, MD

The whole structure of modern medicine is based on four pitifully flawed assumptions.

The first is what I consider to be the greatest tragedy in medical history: the assumption or unspoken premise that "dry mouth" is the only sign of the body's water needs. The whole structure of modern medicine is built on this incorrect and, for want of a stronger word, moronic, assumption that brings about painful premature death to so many millions of people. They suffer because they do not know they are only thirsty.

The human body uses a different logic to the basic "dry mouth" premise that is the cornerstone and very foundation of "modern medical science": to be prepared for the act of chewing and swallowing food, and to facilitate and lubricate this primary function, ample saliva is produced, even if the rest of the body is short of water. In any case, water is too important to the body to only signal its shortage by experiencing a dry mouth.

The second false assumption is that water has no chemical properties of its own and is merely a solvent, a packing material and a means of transporting the ingredients it dissolves. In fact, water is the primary energizer of all functions in the body. It manufactures hydroelectric energy at the cell membranes all over the body, particularly in the neurotransmitter systems. Through its hydrolytic properties, it also and initially breaks down all elements to their primary constituents for absorption into the system for further use, for example, proteins to amino acids, starch to sugar, and fats to fatty acids. In the process, water transfers its hydrolytic energy to these elements that the body can use. Water is also the adhesive that bonds cell membranes. Water, therefore, plays an all-encompassing role in energy metabolism and the physiologic functions of the body.

The third wrong assumption on which modern medicine is built is the thought that because water is free and readily available, there is no reason why the human body should ever become dehydrated. On the contrary, it is easy to become dehydrated even when water is plentiful and has no cost. Studies have shown that as we age, our senses lose their perceptive capabilities. Thus, we gradually lose our ability to realize we are thirsty, and we become more and more dehydrated the older we get.

The fourth false assumption—and one that is encouraged by beverage makers—is the belief that the water needs of the body can be satisfied by any of the commercially prepared fluids. Caffeinated and alcoholic beverages have a dehydrating effect on human physiology. They get more water out of the body than there is water in the cup of beverage or the can of soda.

These mistakes in medical thinking have given birth to the self-expanding "sick-care system" that survives and thrives on people being sick.

My over 20 years of clinical and scientific research has made it clear that the human body has many distinct ways of showing its general or local water needs. Depending on where there is water shortage, many localized complications such as the major pains of the body, or the drought management programs of the body such as asthma, allergies, hypertension and even the autoimmune diseases such as lupus, diabetes, slow viral diseases like chronic fatigue syndrome, and more, are produced.

I believe this information has been methodically and fraudulently concealed until now. My research has now revealed a pleasantly simple and natural cure for many painful and serious health problems. I have called it the "WATER CURE."

The "health-care system" fraud that has thrived on treating dehydration, its manifestation, and adaptive processes with chemicals and procedures has devastated our society. It has caused unnecessary human suffering, on top of burdening people with ever escalating "sick-care" costs.

Enlightened researchers and writers are now trying to intervene and inform the public about chronic dehydration being the primary cause of most of their health problems. Steve Meyerowitz, the seasoned author of this book, has eloquently engaged in bringing this good news to his readers. Fortunately, we are now in a position to prevent, and even cure and eradicate, many of the health problems, at no cost.

All we have to do is to inform people with health problems that they should try water and salt as natural medications since they may not be sick—they may only be manifesting symptoms and signs of thirst and regional drought in the body. Information on the recently uncovered symptoms and signals of chronic, unintentional dehydration is now available. Everyone who taps into this information will be converted into a healer. It is available in this well prepared book, and in the referenced sources used to put this book together.

Readers of this eye-opening publication are encouraged to read further to find more information on health problems, including cancer, associated with unintentional water deficiency in the body. In 1987, as a guest lecturer at an international cancer conference, I provided molecular explanation of how and why unintentional dehydration, in the "fourth dimension of time," is the primary cause of cancer formation in the body. My article, "Pain: A Need for Paradigm Change," was published in the *Journal of Anticancer Research, Sept.-Oct. 1987.*

Dehydration impacts four primary functions of the body that ultimately render it weaker and susceptible to diseases and cancers. Dehydration renders the immune system ineffective and unresponsive. It causes the destruction of some primary amino acids as antioxidants when toxic waste builds up in the body. Some of these amino acids are involved in the enzyme systems that recognize and repair the genetic damage and incorrect DNA transcriptions. The loss of essential amino acids and elements force the cells in a drought stricken area to lose sophistication of function and become primitive and selfish, with self-replicating properties. Dehydration will also cause low-oxygen and high acidity environments that are more suited for cancer cell development than the original normal tissues.

Today, as indicated in this book, a number of research results show increased water intake has strong cancer-preventing effects in the body. It is now up to you to not only read further on the topic, you must make sure your body does not become unintentionally dehydrated. The price you pay for this oversight is enormous.

Dehydration also impacts the molecular metabolism of the body. To treat an already occurring disease, such as cancer, you also need to know what other elements should be added to your diet to reverse the disease process.

God be with you

F. Batmanghelidj, M.D.

Dr. F. Batmanghelidj, MD is author of *Your Body's Many Cries for Water, ABC of Asthma Allergies & Lupus, Water: Rx for A Healthier Pain-Free Life,* and other books and tapes. To learn more about Dr. Batmanghelidj's work, you can visit him at *www.WaterCure.com*.

The Importance of Water in Human Health

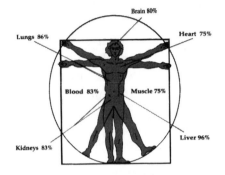

We love water. We play in it, spend our leisure time around it, build our most luxurious homes next to it, enjoy some of our favorite sports on it, exercise in it, travel to exotic vacation spots to be near it, cleanse ourselves with it, and visit spas to seek out its healing powers. We cherish our freshwater lakes, streams, reservoirs, and our great oceans. Nearly seventy percent of the earth's surface is covered with water. And, whether it be by coincidence or divine, our human bodies are also nearly seventy percent water and the salinity of our extracellular fluids is also approximately that of ocean water. These three simple atoms, H_2O, are so integral to our existence, that the discovery of it on another celestial body is almost a certain indicator of life.

The therapeutic use of water in all of its forms crosses all cultures and dates back to the beginning of civilization. The Egyptians, Assyrians, Babylonians, Persians, Greeks, Hebrews, Hindus, Chinese, and Native Americans, all used water to heal injury and treat disease. And here is something else to ponder: The water we drink today is the same water that our ancient ancestors drank. It is the same water that Moses lifted to his lips; that was served to Cleopatra, and to George Washington. The way our ecosystem works, the water on the planet continuously recycles. When sea water evaporates, it leaves the salts behind. As the rising water cools, it condenses to form water droplets and clouds which, at the right temperature, drop back to earth (natural distillation). The same molecules of water are merely exchanged between sea and sky and soil and have been doing so for millennia.

The restorative powers of water are so primal that even the sound of water is healing. CD and audio cassettes of recorded rivers and ocean waves and waterfalls are sold everywhere and there are even videos of them. It is easier to fall asleep or to meditate listening to water. Water is also a fantastic stress reducer. A hot bath before bedtime is the universal cure for relieving the stress that causes insomnia. Special water wands can massage you in the shower and tubs with water jets soothe overstressed areas in your neck, back, and shoulders.

Let's face it, we love water because we are water. The average adult contains 40-50 quarts—10-13 gallons of water! Blood is 83% water, muscles 75%, brain 75%, heart 75%, bones 22%, lungs 86%, kidneys 83%, and eyes 95%.[1] If aliens landed tomorrow, they would probably describe us as mobile sacks of water.

What Does Water Do?

Every cell in every living thing, whether plants or people, contains a nutrient fluid that is mostly water. Every cell is also floating around other cells in an "extracellular" sea of saline water. If the water table for either of these fluids is even slightly under, it

---

Functions of Water in the Human Body

- Improves oxygen delivery to the cells
- Transports nutrients
- Enables cellular hydration
- Moistens oxygen for easier breathing
- Cushions bones and joints
- Absorbs shocks to joints and organs
- Regulates body temperature
- Removes wastes
- Flushes toxins
- Prevents tissues from sticking
- Lubricates joints
- Improves cell to cell communications
- Maintains normal electrical properties of cells
- Empowers the body's natural healing process

is like farmland that is under-irrigated. True, most vegetables will still grow, but they are not in their prime and there are areas of decay. Just look at dry skin to get an idea of what's going on when it's too dry inside you. Where you see shriveled skin, there are shriveled cells. It is like parched soil, only in people, it is one step closer to mummification. You cannot see dehydration, but it is crucial you do not ignore it.

These extracellular fluids carry the electric charges that enable the cells to communicate with each other. They transport food (nutrients), deliver oxygen, and remove the bad stuff—waste products and toxins. They regulate temperature and prevent sticking. On a larger scale this extracellular fluid acts as a lubricant and even a cushion for joints and bones. It acts as a shock absorber for organs and glands. It quenches free radicals by binding to them and is crucial to the body's overall capacity to repair, restore, and heal.

The Dehydration Epidemic

Your body is approximately 67% water by weight. If your body's water content drops by as little as 2%, you will feel fatigued. If it drops by 10%, you will experience significant health problems. Losses greater than that can be fatal. Still, Americans don't drink enough water. In a survey of 3,003 persons in 15 major American cities, participants reported drinking an overall average of only 4.6 eight-ounce servings of water per day compared to the

---

What America Drinks[3]
Servings per day in order of quantity

- Water — 4.6
- Coffee — 1.8
- Milk — 1.3
- Juices — 1.4
- Soda with caffeine — 1.3

- Tea — 1.0
- Soda without caffeine-0.6
- Beer — 0.5
- Wine or other alcoholic beverage — 0.3

The 10 Commandments of Good Hydration

❶ Drink ½ ounce daily for every pound you weigh. A 150lb person drinks 75 ounces, or approximately 2.5 quarts. One glass every hour is a good rule of thumb.

❷ Avoid diuretic beverages that flush water out of your body, such as caffeinated coffee, tea, soda pop, alcohol or beer.

❸ Drink more water and fresh juices to maintain hydration during illness and upon recovery. Illness robs your body of water.

❹ Start your day with ½ to 1 quart of water to flush your digestive tract and rehydrate your system from the overnight fast.

❺ Drink water at regular intervals throughout the day. Don't wait until you're thirsty. Thirst indicates an already present deficiency.

❻ Get in the habit of carrying a water bottle with you or keep one in the car or on your desk. Convenience helps. Stuff it in your shoulder bag or waist pack water bottle pocket. Hiking suppliers have a nice selection of water-bearing belt packs and accessories.

❼ Make a habit of drinking water. According to a survey, the reason most people don't drink as much as they know they ought to, is lack of time or being too busy. Decide to drink water before every meal. Set objectives for yourself such as drinking before you leave the house, and first thing upon your return, or before you start work. Take water breaks instead of coffee breaks. Fill a size glass you can finish or gauge yourself by the number of water bottles you drink during the day.

❽ Increase your drinking when you increase your mental activity level; your stress level; your exercise level.

❾ Drink the purest water available.

❿ Perspire. Exercise to the point of perspiration or enjoy a steam bath. Sweat cleans the lymphatic system and bloodstream. It is one of the best detoxification avenues available to us. Do sweat and do drink plenty of water afterwards to replace the loss of fluids. Drink more in hot weather.

recommended eight servings per day. Forty-four percent said they drank three or less servings per day. Nearly 10% said they didn't drink water at all. Thirty-five percent of Americans are unaware of the number of recommended daily water servings.[2] The survey clearly demonstrates the need for much more public education about the benefits of adequate hydration. The lack of information about proper hydration is worrisome because even minor dehydration can cause problems. Hydration is fast becoming a public health issue that demands greater attention.[3]

Hydration vs. Dehydration

Although Americans drink many liquids, a significant proportion of those fluids are actually dehydrating. We consume 7.9 servings of hydrating beverages each day, but we also drink 4.9 servings of dehydrating beverages, resulting in a net gain of only three hydrating beverages per day. The hydrating and dehydrating drinks cancel each other out. Tap water, bottled water, juice, milk, and carbonated soda without caffeine are all hydrating beverages. Coffee, tea, carbonated soda with caffeine, beer, wine, and other alcoholic drinks are diuretics, meaning they increase the discharge of fluids.

Significant numbers of Americans know little about dehydration. Twenty percent are unaware that coffee and beer are dehydrating. The popularity of bottled water is undermined by the 5 daily servings of diuretic caffeine and alcohol. Once we sum up the total of hydrating and dehydrating beverages, Americans come up dry.

Caffeinated soft drinks are a major offender. Carbonated soft drinks account for more than 27 percent of beverage consumption in the U.S. The average adult American drinks 54.5 gallons of soft drinks per year. In 1997, Americans spent over $54 billion buying soft drinks. For every 16-ounce bottle of water consumed, Americans drank the equivalent of 64 ounces of soda.[4] Carbonated drinks are also the single biggest source of refined sugars in the American diet. It is not much more than liquid candy and 24% of the sodas sold are artificially sweetened.[5] In 1999, the fastest growing soft drink was *Mountain Dew,* which is the brand with the highest caffeine content. We need to look at caffeine for what it really is—a widely used, mildly addictive, psychoactive drug. In large quantity, it can cause restlessness, insomnia, or irregular heartbeat, not to mention disqualification from the Olympics.

What is dehydration? Most people think dehydration is something you get from heat exhaustion. This is when your output of water exceeds your intake. This and dry mouth are the extreme cases. Hidden dehydration is when there is not an adequate amount of water reaching the cells. This mild dehydration can lead to dizziness, lethargy, headache, muscle cramps, loss of appetite, depression and mental fuzziness. We lose water every day through urine, skin (perspiration), feces, and lungs (moist gases). But we also increase our excretion of water by drinking alcohol, beer, coffee, tea, caffeinated cola drinks, and taking some drugs. All are diuretics. Americans drink an average of two cans of soft drinks and two cups of coffee daily. Throw in a few beers in the evening and we are begging for the symptoms of hidden dehydration. Alternatives exist. Instead of taking coffee each morning in order to wake up, try splashing cold water on your face. It is a healthier and more effective wake-up.

Perspiration—Natural Air Conditioning

We lose approximately 2-3 quarts of water every day through the normal vapor exchange through our skin, otherwise known as perspiration. Perspiration is the air conditioning of the body. Without it, we would overheat! You don't have to come off an arduous tennis match to sweat. Perspiration happens even for white collar workers. (Just look at the sales of underarm deodorants.) But that two quarts climbs up to three or four quarts should you play that game of tennis or engage in any other exercise or sport. Those 10-12 cups of water we lose daily need to be replaced to maintain a healthy fluid balance.

How Much to Drink?

You know the food pyramid. It is the chart designed by the National Institute of Health that prioritizes the foods we should eat. The pyramid was redesigned in the 1990s placing fruits and vegetables at the base. Here is a prediction. The next redesign will have eight glasses of water at the pyramid's foundation.

The average adult should drink from 2–3½ quarts of high quality, pure water daily. But the actual amount needs to be customized. It depends on body size, climate, temperature, humidity, altitude of your region, and your exercise level. Even mental activity, stress, and the environment are factors. When you are sick and have a fever, you need more water. Athletes lose fluids fastest. Runners, cyclists, marathoners, etc. should drink before, during, and after their sport. A tennis player who perspires heavily during his game, should drink a pint of water before, during, and after the game. One guide is to take your weight and divide it in half. The resulting number is the amount of ounces you should drink. Thus, a 200 lb person should drink 100 ounces of water daily. If you are drinking an adequate amount, your urine color and odor will be neutral. Don't want to carry around a measuring cup? Just drink from water bottles. Four half-liter water bottles is approximately two quarts (or 2 liters). Finish all by the end of the day. By the way, one sip is one ounce.

What and When to Drink

Do other liquids count as water? Fresh squeezed fruit and vegetable juices are the best alternative to water. Bottled juices are next best. Keep in mind that bottled fruit juices such as apple and orange juice contain large amounts of sugar and that excess sugar causes problems. Non-caffeinated, herbal teas are also an excellent source of water—peppermint, chamomile, licorice, etc. Milks and non-dairy milks such as soy, oat, and rice milks also contribute to your total water intake. Fresh fruits and vegetables also provide water. Diuretic beverages such as alcohol, coffee and caffeinated teas, and soft drinks, do not count. They have the opposite effect of drawing water out of the body.

If we assume the average person needs to imbibe four half liters of water daily (about 2 quarts), then here is one possible way to break it up. Drink one half liter in the morning before breakfast. This is a great flush of your intestines and helps prepare the stomach for food and avoids constipation. Next take another half liter before lunch, another before dinner, and finally another by bedtime. Always drink before meals (15-20 minutes before) or 1-3 hours after meals. Too much water during a meal dilutes your digestive enzymes. Too much water on a full stomach flushes the stomach contents before digestion is complete. If water is not conveniently available between meals, eat fresh fruit. Don't wait until you are thirsty to have a drink. By the time your body signals for more water, you are already behind in your water needs. Drink extra on airplanes where the atmosphere is as dry as a desert. Water also reportedly reduces the severity of jet lag.

Essentials of Rehydration

❶ Drink enough to equal 1/2 your body weight in ounces, daily. Thus, if you weigh 200 lbs, drink 100 ounces.
❷ Use 1/4 tsp. of sea salt for every quart of water you drink. Use salt generously with food, as long as you drink enough water.
❸ Avoid diuretics, such as caffeinated or alcoholic drinks. Every six oz. of caffeine or alcohol requires an additional 10 to 12 oz. of water to rehydrate you.

Keep water handy. Insulated quart size cups and belt packs with water bottle holders are available in sports stores. Avoid drinking ice water. Your body has to produce more heat to neutralize those icy temperatures. Ice cold temperatures shock the stomach during which time it cannot secret enzymes. Cold water is fine; it is cooling, especially to an overheated body, but ice water, because of its extreme temperature, is undesirable.

Sodium and Potassium

Sodium is arguably the most important mineral in the body. The extracellular fluid is a saline solution. Salt is necessary to maintain normal osmotic pressure for the transport of nutrients and waste to and from the cells. It also facilitates hydroelectric activity (communications) from cell to cell. Salt retains water and thus is a buffer against dehydration. Sodium also enables ATP generation. ATP supplies energy to cells and muscles. Athletes who push their bodies longer than five hours, especially in hot weather, run the risk of using up their sodium and their water before anything else.

In 1982, Alberto Salazar won the Boston Marathon and proceeded immediately to the emergency room at Boston Hospital to receive six liters of intravenous solution to replenish his lost water and salt. Why? He overheated. These marathoners demonstrate the basic daily requirements of the human body that are normally invisible to us. In a study of 64 athletes at an ironman race lasting between 9 and 15 hours, 27 percent were hyponatremic (salt deficient) and 17 percent of them needed medical attention.[6] This suggests that athletes should aim for 80 to 100 mg sodium per quart of water.

"Chronic cellular dehydration of the body is the primary etiology of painful, degenerative diseases."
—F. Batmanghelidj, M.D

Potassium is mostly present in intracellular fluid. Its main role is the regulation of total body water and stabilizing muscle contractions. This is the key mineral that is lost through sweat and urine. In a study of athletes running 40 minutes at 70 degrees Fahrenheit, potassium loss was estimated at 435 mg/hour or 200 mg per kg of weight lost.[7] Supplementing with potassium during exercise increases muscle hydration.[8]

Dr. Batmanghelidj and Salt

Dr. F. Batmanghelidj is the world's leading hydration crusader. His book, *Your Body's Many Cries for Water,*[9] affixes the blame for a host of modern ailments on the lack of proper hydration. In his theory, water and salt follow oxygen as the most crucial ingredients for life. Proper hydration can reverse and improve a wide range of

health problems such as allergies, asthma, hypertension, choles-
terol, premature aging, Alzheimer's, back pain, migraine head-
aches, obesity, and depression. A medical doctor himself,
Batmanghelidj reminds us that one of the first protocols for a
patient upon hospitalization is an intravenous saline solution.
Doctors are well aware that dehydration, second only to oxygen
deprivation, robs life fastest. Minor dehydration—not enough to
kill—is both the result and the hidden cause of many illnesses. The
inverse is also true. Good hydration is at the foundation of good
health. Drink up now, because the price for administering an
intravenous saline water solution in the hospital is approximately
$350.

Early Signs of Dehydration	Mature Signals of Dehydration[10]	Signs of Emergency Dehydration
Fatigue	Heartburn	Asthma and Allergies
Anxiety	Joint and back pain	Old Age Diabetes
Irritability	Migraine Headaches	Hypertension
Depression	Fibromyalgia	Autoimmune
Cravings	Constipation/colitis	Diseases, Lupus,
Cramps	Anginal pain	Psoriasis, etc.
Headache		

From Dr. Batmanghelidj's perspective, most so-called incur
able diseases are nothing more than disease labels given to various
stages of drought. Americans diligently check the fluids in their
cars, but neglect the fluids in their bodies. In a car, oil prevents
metal from rubbing up against metal. In the body, water keeps
cartilage robust and joints floating. Once dehydration sets in,
cartilage thins and fails to buffer the joints and bone rubs against
bone causing arthritic pain. But doctors are not taught to check the
water and salt levels. Instead they treat the complaint with pain
killers that mask the body's alert signals.[10] Pain killers treat the
effect, not the cause, and eventually surgeons shave off some bone
to create more float in the joint or replace the joint altogether.
Taking a pain killer in this instance is like cutting the wires to stop
the oil light in your car from flashing. If auto mechanics used the
same logic as mainstream medicine, they would never check the

fluids and when things wore out, they would simply install replacement parts.

There are two kinds of water in the body: Intracellular and extracellular—inside the cells and surrounding the cells. To the degree that water can reach every cell, the cell can be regularly cleansed and the waste products of normal cell metabolism can be carried away. Once inside the cells, the water is held there by potassium. Batmanghelidj says there are two oceans of water in the body, intracellular and extracellular. The saline content of the water outside the cells is said to be similar to the saline content of the ocean. Good health depends on maintaining the balance between these two internal oceans. The balance is achieved by regular intake of water, potassium from the diet, and salt. When there is insufficient water to reach the cells, they draw upon the extracellular water. This is the first stage of dehydration. It is also the cause of edema because the brain commands an increase in salt in order to retain more water. When the shortage of water reaches a more critical level, the body increases the osmotic pressure in order to deliver more water to the cells. This is a cause of hypertension.[11]

Within the three months that I have been drinking the right amount of water the right way, my chronic mucous began to leave, my hair became soft, and my skin is becoming softer. I have fewer wrinkles (I am almost 70 years old). My stomach aches stopped. My toenails are not brittle. Two black spots I have had on my leg from several years ago as an aftermath of deep cuts have disappeared. My eyebrows grew back. There are dark streaks showing in my gray hair. My hair is coming in thicker and my memory is improving.
—Ann Louise Gittleman, author *Guess What Came to Dinner.*[12]

Increasing the intake of your water must be slow and spaced out until there is a corresponding excretion of urine. When the urine is clear, it indicates we are drinking adequate amounts of water. Salt is also lost in the urine which helps get rid of edema.

Water is arguably our best diuretic. For years mainstream medicine has preached the avoidance of salt because it promotes high blood pressure and salt has become taboo. But this boomerang reaction of avoiding salt can backfire on our health. The proper proportion of salt to water, ¼ teaspoon per quart of water, is necessary to maintain proper hydration and to generate hydroelectric energy needed for cell to cell communication—the spark of life. If your weight suddenly increases, you are taking too much salt. The cure?—Drink more water.

To learn more about salt, water, and potassium and how to balance them to treat autoimmune diseases such as lupus, chronic fatigue, psoriasis, etc., and allergies, asthma, edema, hypertension, and other diseases, see Dr. Batmanghelidj's books listed in the resource chapter.

After only four days of drinking eight glasses of water, eight year old Jeremy's asthma cleared up to the extent that he was able to discontinue all of his medications. Within one month his lung capacity increased from 60% of normal to 120%. Arthritis, ulcers, edema, even blood pressure—I've seen them all improve with water.
—Julian Whitaker, M.D., editor Health & Healing Newsletter

Asthma, Allergies, and Dehydration

Asthma is the constriction of the air sacs in the lungs. Histamine is an important neurotransmitter that regulates the body's thirst mechanism and water intake. In a condition of dehydration, histamine production increases, which in turn swells the body tissues, including the small sacs of the lungs. This constricts the air flow causing the tell-tale shortness of breath experienced in asthma. Allergies and asthma cause histamine to be released because histamine is part of the body's immune response. Dehydration would ordinarily cause dryness in the membranes of the nose and eyes, but histamine and its subordinate chemicals increase the distribution of water to those organs.

Today there are more than 25 different anti-histamine drugs available for treating asthma and allergies. However, according to Batmanghelidj, dehydration is one of the causes of histamine release. In fact, the inverse is also true, water and salt are two very strong, natural anti-histamines. For an asthma or allergy attack, he recommends drinking 3-4 glasses of water followed by a few grains of salt on the tongue. As a preventative, the asthma and allergy patient should force themselves to drink the recommended amount of water daily to avoid excessive histamine release.[13]

Cancer Protection from Water?

It is a little known fact, but insufficient water consumption is actually a risk factor for getting colon, breast, and urinary tract cancers such as cancers of the kidneys, bladder, prostate, and testicles. When the body is well hydrated, blood circulation is expanded and immune system cells can reach the cancerous tissues in greater numbers. Statistical studies indicate that cancer victims drink precious little of the wet stuff. On the other hand, women who drink more than five glasses of water per day actually reduce their chance of getting kidney and bladder cancer by 45 percent. Men reduce their chances of contracting prostate and testicle cancer by 32 percent.[14] How can this be? The theory is that water flushes toxins from the body before they can do their damage or be reabsorbed. In one study, female water drinkers reduced their risk of developing breast cancer by 79%. One interpreter of the study, water expert Dr. Susan M. Kleiner, postulates that "possibly maintaining a dilute solution within the cells reduces the potency of estrogen and its ability to cause hormone-related cancer."[15]

Kidney stones affect approximately 15% of the population and kidney stone manufacture can be another side effect of insufficient water consumption. One study reported that individuals with a history of kidney stones reduced their reoccurrence by as much as 15% just by increasing their water intake to 4 or more glasses per day. Lack of water promotes the formation of the stones by concentrating the calcium salts inside the kidneys.

Lose Weight with Water

Are you thirsty or hungry? It is possible that we are interpreting our signs of thirst for hunger. Food is a major source of water and about one third of our daily water intake comes from foods. Raw fruits and vegetables are 70% to 95% water. Even bread is 35% water. So it is possible that your desire for food is a hidden

---

How Much Water for How Much Food?

More than 80% of the water consumed in the US goes to animals and agriculture. Below is the number of gallons it takes to deliver a serving of the following foods to your dinner table.

2,607 gallons	Steak	26 gallons	Dinner Roll
408 gallons	Chicken	12 gallons	Baked Potato
100 gallons	Pat of butter		

---

desire for water. Try not eating between meals. Reach for the water bottle instead of the ice cream. Once you fill up on water, it creates a satiety—a feeling of fullness. Then get busy with something. Chances are your mind will be off your stomach; you will feel full, and your hunger will disappear. Repeat this daily and you will save calories and shed pounds. Sometimes hunger masquerades as thirst.

The Fountain of Youth

According to legend, the fountain of youth is a spring of water located on a Bahamian island. This is the spring for which Ponce de León earnestly searched. This island, surrounded by its green ocean, blue sky, and pristine air, is in itself a healing experience. But drinking its healing waters was purported to rejuvenate the drinker. All around the earth, one can find healing waters, from steam baths to mineral spas, to geysers and springs, these waters are some of the most special places on earth. The stuff that comes out is truly God's liquid.

Can water keep you young? There is a theory that cells are immortal and just the fluids in and around them degenerates over time. If you subscribe to this theory, then replenishing them with adequate amounts of the highest quality water is the simplest and most sublime way to stave off the process of aging. The stooping of older people, their dry wrinkled skin, and brittle bones all point to a dehydrated condition. But this condition did not occur overnight. This dehydration, as well as that of other illnesses, is a chronic condition that accumulates for years until your "thirst" manifests itself in pain. Water is the most important element in your body. Your cells cannot function without it. Low level dehydration can be both perfectly hidden and managed. The body simply adapts to a state of drought. But this condition manifests many long-term illnesses which shorten our lives and eventually cripple our health.

"The cell is immortal. It is merely the fluid in which it floats that degenerates." –Dr. Alexis Carrel, French-born American surgeon and biologist and winner of the 1912 Nobel Prize

---

Hydrotherapy - The Curative Powers of Water

While water cannot be described as a magic potion, it has enormous curative powers. Anyone who has ever visited a Roman bath, a steam bath, or jumped into a jaquzzi or a whirlpool knows the power of water. Mud baths, sitz baths, mineral salt baths, enemas, douches, even swims in the ocean are healing and invigorating. Witness the yearly pilgrimage of millions of people who flock to the Dead Sea to swim in its healing, highly saline waters.

Therapeutically, hot water soothes and relaxes the body, and because it releases tension in the nerves, it can have reflexive action to nearly every organ of the body. Dry heat is simply not as penetrating as wet heat. According to Dr. Douglas Lewis, N.D., Chairperson of Physical Medicine at the Bastyr College Natural Health Clinic in Seattle, Washington, external applications of hot water work because they produce "a response that stimulates the immune system and cause white cells to migrate out of the blood vessels and into the tissues where they clean up toxins and assist the body in eliminating wastes." Cold water discourages inflammation by constricting blood vessels (vasoconstriction), and reduces inflammatory agents such as histamine. Dr. Lewis cautions that short cold water treatment may actually increase fever and only long cold water treatment pulls heat from the body for fever reduction.[16]

Hydrotherapy is not just alternative medicine. Mainstream orthopedists already recommend water therapy after hip, knee, and joint surgery and the first thing any doctor recommends after injury is ice. Underwater movement relieves stress on joints and also has aerobic benefits. Runners sometimes practice running underwater. Cold water also enhances muscle tone. And there are numerous cardiovascular and muscular benefits to underwater exercises because of its inherent resistance.

Alternating between hot and cold water reduces inflammation and congestion, and stimulates the adrenals and endocrine glands. According to Leon Chaitow, N.D., D.O., of London, England, hot and cold water therapy improves circulation, especially to the digestive areas, and improves the detoxifying capacity of the liver.[17] So, next time you have a tummy ache, resist reaching for the Digel or Tums. Place a hot water bottle on the stomach and rest. When you are fatigued, just slide into a hot bath. External hydrotherapy is safe, natural, inexpensive, and an effective home treatment for many common health conditions that can keep the doctor away.

What's Wrong with Our Drinking Water?

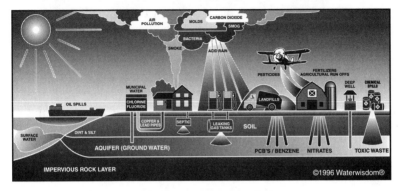

The Evolution of Pollution: From factory and farm to stream and soil.

One hundred years ago, people died from drinking contaminated water. Cholera, diarrhea, hookworm, trichuriasis, were all traced to water. With an increase in the population and the demand for water, came an increase in water's contaminants. Our municipalities have the enormous job of purifying the tremendous volume of water that flows into our homes. Americans feel there is an abundant, never-ending supply of pure drinking water. Yet, when we turn on the tap, only two percent of the water that pours out is ever used for cooking and drinking. In fact, we live in one of the few countries in the world where you can drink from the garden hose without worry. Even the water used to flush the toilet is pure enough to drink. Sadly, our aging water treatment and distribution systems were not built to handle modern-day contaminants. Nor can our aging water treatment plants keep up with our ever expanding population and it would take billions of dollars to upgrade them.

Current *Environmental Protection Agency* (EPA) guidelines allow for "acceptable" levels of pollutants, such as chlorine, lead, arsenic, and aluminum in our water. But even with these less than stringent EPA treatment standards, the 1993 and 1994 EPA reports indicate that some 53 million Americans drank from city water systems that violated EPA standards. In 1995, it was officially recommended by the EPA that people with compromised immune systems due to AIDS, chemotherapy, or transplant surgery boil their water or use bottled water.[18]

Some experts claim that even all the measures we currently have in place do not insure a pure drinking water supply. The question facing the public is: if our municipal treatment plants cannot produce contaminant-free water, what can be done to create healthy drinking water?

The Challenge for Municipal Water Treatment Plants

It is true that tap water is mostly free of bacteria and parasites thanks to chlorination. But bacteria represent only a fraction of the modern-day hazards present in our water. The nation's 50,000 municipal water supplies are liberally laced with hundreds of potentially harmful substances that have long-term ramifications for our health. According to the *Center for Disease Control* (CDC) in Atlanta, nearly

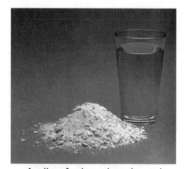

A pile of mineral scale and pollutants from tap water.

one million people get sick from drinking contaminated water each year with about 1,000 of those cases ending in fatalities.

There are more than 75,000 chemical compounds in our water with more being added daily. They come from industry, agriculture, and consumers/homes. Small doses of them in drinking water are ingested every day and no one knows what their long-term effect will be. Even our modern technology is no match for testing these many pollutants, much less eliminating them.

The Pollutants

Landfills are still a major source of groundwater contamination in spite of new regulations. Industrial waste and municipal sewage continue to make their way into our waterways. Cesspools, septic systems, underground storage tanks, and lawn treatments all runoff into our water. Rain and snow also help pollutants and pesticides in the air find their way into the water. Runoff from pesticides or nitrates from nitrogen fertilizer plague water supplies in agricultural areas. Even radioactive waste finds its way into our environment as a result of inadequate disposal procedures and enforcement.

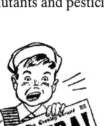

Gasoline & MTBE

We use a lot of gasoline in this country. Any seepage, leaks, spills, or accidents lead to contamination. Gasoline hangs out on sediment and contaminates

The headlines about contaminated water problems are just as frequent today as they were at the start of the Clean Water Act in the 1970s.

runoff water or water flowing through filtering beds on its way to underground aquifers. One gallon of gasoline ruins 5 million gallons of drinking water. There are thousands of underground gasoline storage tanks that still remain in the ground beyond their twenty year life expectancy.

MTBE is a gasoline additive that has been used since 1980 to limit gasoline's air pollution. Experiments demonstrate that laboratory rats and mice who breathe or drink it develop lymphoma, leukemia, testicular, thyroid, and kidney tumors. According to a U.S. Geological Survey and the Department of Environmental Study at Oregon Institute, MTBE has contaminated about one-third of the nation's drinking wells in 31 states. In California, about 10,000 groundwater sites have been found to contain MTBE. In Texas, over 21,000 storage tanks have been found to be leaking with MTBE traced to 12 municipal water supplies. Government response to MTBE seems inadequate given that the *Leaking Underground Storage Tanks Program* is said to have a backlog of 168,900 tanks.[19] MTBE is not biodegradable and has been called the "biggest environmental crisis of the decade" by the CBS news program *60 Minutes*. California Senator Barbara Boxer called on the EPA to investigate reports that the oil industry knew about MTBE threats to drinking water before the controversial gasoline additive was introduced.

Parasites

The CDC estimates about 900,000 cases each year of water-borne bacterial disease. Even though many municipal supplies have been treated according to the *Safe Drinking Water Act,* millions of Americans are still wary of drinking tap water. After all, as many as one-third of all gastrointestinal illnesses are said to be caused by bacterial and parasitic infections as well as 900 deaths each year.

Cryptosporidium is a kind of parasite that causes acute and chronic cases of diarrhea, cramps, fever, and vomiting. Because it is only 5 microns in size—250 of them can fit on the head of a pin—it can slip through typical water treatment plants and enter our drinking water. What is more, it is resistant to chlorine. Once ingested, this unicellular parasite hatches eggs in the digestive tract. In 1993, 400,000 people in Milwaukee suffered from cryptosporidium contaminated tap water, and 104 people died.[20]

As few as 30 parasites—one glass of water—can cause long-term infection. In other words, one glass of water can cause long term problems. There is no established cure. Healthy individuals can recover in 1-2 weeks, but crypto can be life-threatening to those with compromised immune systems. About 50% of AIDS patients who contract the parasite die from it. Chemotherapy and organ transplant patients, the elderly and chronically ill, infants and children are all at risk. Distillation and submicron filtration at your tap are currently the best insurance to avoid cryptosporidium.

Another chlorine resistant parasite is the protozoa *Giardia lamblia.* Giardia causes symptoms similar to colitis, irritable bowel syndrome, and lactose intolerance as well as cramps, diarrhea, and nausea. It is often mistaken for other ailments. One to two weeks of antibiotic or herbal antimicrobial therapy is required for recovery. *Escherichia Coli (E. coli)* is a common, nonpathogenic bacteria that resides in our digestive tract and that of animals. Its presence in water is an indication of fecal contamination. E. coli infection from water or food can cause dysentery-like symptoms.

Additives to Water

There are dozens of additives used to treat municipal water. Chlorine and fluoride are the most common and the most infamous. There is a whole category of additives known as flocculents which cause pollutants to clump together for more efficient filtering. Even though the EPA classifies some flocculents as probable human carcinogens, it still allows their use in water treatment facilities.[21]

"It is estimated that in 99 percent of the US population, their fatty tissue contains one or more of the toxic chemicals found in water."—Dr. Ronald Klatz, MD, Pres. American Academy of Anti-Aging Medicine[22]

Chlorine

In the early 1920s, the United States successfully controlled the outbreaks of cholera, typhoid, hepatitis, dysentery, and other waterborne diseases using chlorine. Today, chlorine is still accepted as the only viable method of killing bacteria in water supplies. Ironically, this process that once rid our water of these infectious organisms, is now responsible for causing a new breed of dangerous pollutants.

Historically, chlorine was the world's first biological weapon with its use as poisonous gas in WWI. Later it was drafted for civilian use to poison the bacteria in our water. At its most benign, chlorine makes it seem as if one is drinking from a swimming pool.

But, if the chlorine in water is sufficient to produce an offensive smell, it could be enough to destroy helpful bacteria in our intestinal tract.

But chlorination is responsible for a more insidious problem. It is extremely volatile and combines rapidly with organic, carbon based pollutants from industry and the environment, to form a new breed of dangerous chemicals called tri-halo-methanes (THMs). There are hundreds of deadly THMs, among them carbon-tetrachloride, bis-chloroethane, and chloroform. According to a Norwegian study by Dr. Per Magnus of the *National Institute of Public Health*, Oslo, THMs have mutagenic and carcinogenic effects. Dr. Magnus found that the use of chlorine leads to a 14% increase in overall birth defects. In another study of 5,144 pregnant women conducted by the California Department of Health Services, women who drank five glasses of THM contaminated water had a 16.4% rate of miscarriage as compared to a 6.1% rate of those who had low levels of THMs in their water.[23]

These chemicals plus the larger family of chlorinated hydrocarbons, such as DDT, PCBs, TCE, 2,4,5-T, have been linked to heart disease, senility, and cancers of the bladder, liver, pancreas, colon and urinary tract.

In addition to consuming disinfection byproducts, there is concern that water used in baths, showers, dishwashers and washing machines may contribute in indoor pollution. Chemicals resulting from chlorination of water become airborne when passed through appliances used in the home. When THM contaminated water is used for showers, toxic vapors are easily inhaled.

A new alternative disinfectant, used in many cities, is chloramine—a mix of chlorine and ammonia. Much is unknown about the safety of this disinfectant and there are many concerns such as the ability of aquarium filters in fish tanks and home dialysis machines to remove it.

Hydrocarbons

Hydrocarbons are everywhere. They are the mainstay of the chemical industry and they are both very stable and fat soluble. When they enter our environment, they stay for a long time and are hard to get rid of. Hundreds of millions of tons of hydrocarbon waste are produced in the United States every year. Many make their way into our water supplies through agricultural runoff, industrial effluents, sewage, and chemical dumps. They end up in our rivers, lakes, reservoirs, and groundwater. Hydrocarbons are so insidious, they have made their way into such far-reaching places as the fat of the arctic penguin and human breast tissue.

Upgrading Our Aging Municipal Water Systems

Americans don't trust the water coming out of their taps. Sales of bottled water are so hot, it has become the fastest growing beverage in America. They're right! Municipal water systems need to be significantly upgraded just to meet federal standards. The EPA says 55,000 community water systems will have to be upgraded including the replacement of aging distribution pipes. The cost is over $420 billion and that is only the estimated cost. This is a monumental project that will take decades to complete.

Fluoridation of Municipal Water

Fluoride is without doubt the most controversial ingredient in our water. Since it was first introduced into municipal water supplies in the 1940s, it has been the subject of a heated battle between established medical associations, scientists, researchers, politicians, and consumer groups. Some 130 million people living in this country drink fluoridated water. Fluoride has been banned in Sweden, Denmark, and Holland, and abandoned in Belgium and West Germany. America has not budged in its loyalty to fluoride, yet our rate of tooth decay is among the highest in the world. On the other hand, there are many nations that are not fluoridated, yet largely decay free. The Otomi Indians in Mexico, the Bedouins in Israel, and the Ibos in Nigeria are all primitive societies with no fluoride and no tooth decay. Why? Because they consume almost no refined carbohydrates and sugar.[24]

The idea for adding fluoride to the nation's water supplies was first proposed in 1939 by Dr. Gerald Cox of the Mellon Institute, a research organization that is funded by the Mellon family, owners of Alcoa Aluminum. Fluoride is a waste product of the aluminum industry. Their research showed that fluoride in drinking water accumulated in teeth and made the tooth enamel more insoluble thus reducing the incidence of cavities.

Most major medical organizations in the country continue to support mass fluoridation: *The American Medical Association, the American Dental Association,* and the federal government's *U.S. Public Health Service.* One defection from the ranks is the *Worcester Dental Society,* who repudiated its own endorsement of fluoridation. The society said that its endorsement had been given after having heard only one side that relied on tests "of an unscientific nature" conducted in the 1940s, and reported on by the aluminum trust. They further stated that fluoride does not prevent tooth decay and that better nutrition, hygiene and supervision were the cause of the benefits attributed to fluoride.[25]

Physicians Desk Reference - Side Effects of Fluoride

- Dental fluorosis (mottling of the teeth)
- Skin eruptions (such as eczema)
- Gastric distress
- Immune system problems
- Down's Syndrome (genetic damage)
- Breakdown of collagen protein
- Heart problems
- Headache

Why the controversy? The answers lie in the fact that fluoride is a known poison. In concentrated form, it has been used as a rat poison, a pesticide, and for deworming pigs and delousing chickens. In humans, as little as one-tenth of an ounce will cause death. The adverse effects of fluoride are well documented in the *Physician's Desk Reference (see box).* In *Fluoridation-The Great Dilemma,*

Doctors Waldbott, Burgstahler, and McKinney add to the list: hypothyroidism, kidney disease, diabetes, hypoglycemia, hormonal imbalance, lowered enzyme activity, reduced fertility, birth defects, and cancer.[26]

One of the major complaints about fluoride is that what we are putting into our drinking water is the waste product of the aluminum and phosphate fertilizer industries. ALCOA and others have paid large fines for poisoning animals and vegetation and for improper dumping that has contaminated soil and water.

Benefit to Children?

Children are supposed to benefit most from fluoride's anti-cavity effects. But a 1990s study found that fluoridation does not reduce decay in permanent teeth. The dental records of 39,207 school children, aged 5-17 and from 84 geographical areas throughout the U.S., showed that the number of decayed, missing, and filled permanent teeth per child was 2.0 in fluoridated areas, 2.0 in nonfluoridated areas and 2.2 in partially fluoridated areas.[27] In New Zealand, Canada, and the U.S., other studies by public health dentists have repeated these findings.

After completing his investigation with results similar to the U.S. study, the former Chief Dental Officer of the Department of Health for Auckland, New Zealand, Dr. John Colquhoun, began to campaign against fluoridation. His study, which used statistics on the tooth decay of 60,000 12-13 year olds, also showed that fluoride was damaging teeth in the form of dental fluorosis.[28] This condition when mild, appears as a chalky white area on the tooth; when stronger, the teeth become yellow, brown, or black and the tips break off.

Fluoride affects more than teeth. In two studies in the 1950s, Dr. Lionel Rapaport of the University of Wisconsin, found that fluoridated towns had roughly twice as many Down's Syndrome births as nonfluoridated towns. A 1989 study by Procter and Gamble showed that genetic damage is caused with even half the amount of fluoride normally used in public water supplies.[29]

The 1992 *Canadian Dental Association's* proposed guidelines recommends: "Fluoride supplements should not be recommended for children less than three years old...fluoride damages teeth by interfering with the proper formation of collagen and collagen-like proteins in the tooth during the formative stages. These proteins also comprise the structural component for skin, ligaments, muscles, cartilage, and bone. Fluoridated water leads to a breakdown of these proteins."[30]

The Fluoride - Cancer Link

Fifty thousand fluoridation linked cancer deaths occur yearly in the U.S., according to Dr. Dean Burk, former head chemist of the *National Cancer Institute*. He spoke at an EPA hearing in 1985 imploring an end to the use of fluoride in drinking water. Citing a study of cancer death rates in Birmingham, England, Dr. Burk found that there was a large increase of cancer after only a few years of artificially fluoridating water supplies there.

The *National Cancer Institute*, the *New Jersey Department of Health*, and the *Safe Water Foundation* all found that during the period of 1991-1993, men exposed to fluoridated water had a far higher incidence of osteosarcoma than those who were not. "In human studies, fluoride has been shown to transform white blood cells into cells 'suggestive of reticuloendothelial malignancy.'[31]

In a monumental study released in December of 1975 and read into the Congressional Record, Dr. Burk and Dr. John Yamouyiannis, a biochemist and science director of the National Health Foundation, examined 10 fluoridated and 10 nonfluoridated cities over a 30 year period with corrections for demographic variables such as age, race and sex. The cancers discovered occurred mostly in the gastrointestinal tract, mouth, esophagus, stomach, large intestine and rectum. The report was tested in court by pro-fluoridationists on several occasions, yet according to one of the judges, "Point by point, every criticism...made of the Burk-Yiamouyiannis study was met and explained."[32] According to Dr. Yiamouyiannis, the exact relationship between fluoride and cancer is not known other than that it is a mutagenic substance. This means it changes genetic structure of cell and chromosomes.

The amount of fluoride used to fluoridate public water systems leads to soft tissue fluoride levels which damage biologically important chemicals, such as enzymes, leading to a wide range of diseases. A study published in the *Journal of the American Chemical Society* provided the chemical evidence to support this view."[33]

The U.S. Public Health Service in a 1993 study said: "in cultured human and rodent cells, the weight of the evidence leads to the conclusion that fluoride exposure results in increased chromosome aberrations (genetic damage)."[34]

Other Problems

The *Journal of the American Medical Association* published three articles in 1990, 1991, and 1992 that linked increased hip fracture rates to fluoridated areas. The *New England Journal of Medicine,* also found that "fluoride treatment of osteoporosis causes bone fractures. Osteoporosis is one of the first signs of poisoning due to fluoride in the water. As little as 0.7 ppm fluoride in the water has been associated with skeletal fluorosis."[35]

The use of fluoride is a financial and political issue. Consumer advocate Ralph Nader said that "industrial pressure forced the U.S. Public Health Service to prematurely endorse fluoridation."According to Michael Wollan, author of *Controlling the Potential Hazards of Government Sponsored Technology*, it is difficult for agencies and professional organizations to reverse themselves on a cause they have promoted for years.

Who Do You Believe?

What makes the fluoride issue so confusing is that the public does not know who to believe. Because of blanket endorsements by large established medical organizations, dentists are inundated with pro-fluoridation literature. Findings contrary to accepted policy are suppressed. When such findings are cited, they are rebuked because statistical studies have so many variables, they can be twisted and debunked. But no matter which side you believe, one thing is indisputable—mass fluoridation eliminates our freedom of choice.

Ecological Hazards of Modern Society

Unfortunately, our water is subject to nearly every kind of pollutant in our society. As if contamination from gasoline, parasites, chlorine, fluoride, and aging pipes were not enough, pharmaceutical drugs, pesticides, lead, asbestos, nitrates, and even radioactive waste all have an impact on our water.

Drugs

Watch what you flush down the toilet. A new form of contaminant was recently found in Berlin's tap water. Europeans and Americans are flushing antibiotics along with birth control pills, perfumes, and pain relievers down their toilets. These chemicals pass through old-fashioned wastewater treatment plants and then into rivers, lakes, and aquifers. At the American Chemical Society's annual meeting, Thomas Heberer of the Technical University of Berlin revealed finding high concentrations of chemical fragrances used in perfumes, shampoos, and detergents accumulating in the flesh of perch, carp, and other fish down river from sewage treatment plants in Berlin. Also, sun blocking compounds from sunscreen lotion were found in the flesh of fish and eels. The compounds according to Heberer are "long-lived in water and easily penetrate the cells of aquatic organism."[36]

Heberer and a colleague first found the cholesterol-lowering drug, clofibric acid, while testing for pesticides in groundwater. Then they found it in tap water. According to the U.S. Geological Survey (USGS), other complex drugs, which survive the human digestive system and enter water systems are heart medications, antidepressants, anti-epileptics, anticancer chemicals, sex hormones, antibiotics, hormone replacement, aspirin, vitamins, ibuprofen, and caffeine.

"The body's ability to break down medicine varies widely by individual and drug. Chemotherapy drugs retain nearly all their potency as they leave the body, while female hormones enter the sewage system inert but are reactivated through chemical reactions during treatment."[37]

Antibiotics and hormones from animal feedlots also find their way into waterways from manure and sewage sludge spread on the land. USGS researchers have found a wide variety of antibiotics miles downstream from hog waste lagoons located in North Carolina, Missouri, and Iowa.

Pesticides and Herbicides

If you happen to live in an agricultural based state, chances are fairly strong that your well or public water supply is laced with pesticides or nitrates from nitrogen fertilizer runoff.

A recent report by the *Environmental Working Group* in Washington, DC revealed that over 14 million people living in a 14 state area are drinking water laced with herbicides and pesticides. The herbicides found were used to treat corn and soybeans.[38] Over 67 pesticides have been found in water supplies throughout the Midwest, the Chesapeake Bay region, Louisiana and the District of Columbia. Birth defects, genetic mutations, neurological damage, oxygen starvation, blue baby syndrome, heart and artery disease, and cancer are all worsened by the ingestion of these chemicals.

Quality of Pipes

Over 90% of the water distribution pipes in this country are over 100 years old. Galvanized pipes began to be widely used in the 1920s and copper pipes replaced lead. But a major source of lead contamination today is the lead solder used. It was legal up until 1986 to use lead pipes, lead solder, and other lead materials in water pipe repair and construction. Lead plumbing is therefore ubiquitous and because these pipes are buried underground and hidden behind walls, they are likely to be with us for decades.

Dioxin

Dioxin was developed as a defoliant for use in the Vietnam War and is one of the most deadly chemicals ever made. It was the prime contaminant involved in the infamous Love Canal chemical spill. It never breaks down in the environment.

Acid Rain

The eastern seaboard (including Canada) receives the effects of some 27 million tons of sulfur dioxide and 21 million tons of nitrous oxides a year generated from Midwest smoke stacks. The result: acid rain, snow, dew and fog creating polluted reservoirs and watersheds, dead lakes, damaged crops, and forests of stunted trees. An investigation by the Congressional Office of Technology Assessment in June, 1984, concluded that 17,000 lakes and 112,000 miles of streams are threatened by acid rain creating widespread water pollution and an impending national disaster.[39]

Scientists have known for many years that emissions from factories, cars, smelters, coal, and electric generating plants travel into the atmosphere and make their way back to us with the next rain. This "acid rain" not only damages the quality of our water in lakes and streams, watersheds, and forests, but also harms the fish, wildlife species, and most important of all, human health.

Heavy Metals

Lead. One in six Americans drinks water containing excessive levels of lead, a systemic toxin. The EPA has found that the drinking water in some 130 cities serving 42 million people has lead levels in excess of federal limits. The cities must remedy this, but they have until 2013 to do so. Most cities won't meet this deadline due to lack of funds.

Many older buildings still contain lead pipes and if the pipes are not lead, lead solder was probably used on the joints. The longer water is in contact with lead, the more lead it picks up. Lead will dissolve more readily when water is acidic (having a pH of less than 7.0); and hot water dissolves lead more quickly than cold water. Natural and industrial soil deposits and brass alloy faucets are another source of lead contamination. The disposal of lead paints can further pollute our water supplies. The EPA estimates that lead from drinking water contributes about 20% of the average person's total lead exposure.

Lead can impair the reproductive and central nervous systems and may cause problems with behavioral and emotional development. It can increase blood pressure in adults, and affect hearing. High levels of exposure can cause anemia, kidney damage and mental retardation.

Children absorb a much greater percent of ingested lead than do adults. Bottle-fed infants may absorb as much as 85%. In infants and children, lead causes behavioral problems, learning disabilities, retardation and stunted growth. Studies have shown that continuous small doses of lead from drinking water can lower the intelligence of gifted children to that of normal children, and drop children of normal intelligence to the bottom of their class.

Arsenic. Arsenic occurs widely in the environment from natural sources such as air, water, food, and tobacco, as well as arsenic containing pesticides. Its maximum level is set at 0.05 mg/l. At present it has not been labeled as a definite carcinogen, but it does attack the digestive tract and lungs, and can cause lethargy and fatigue at low levels.

Aluminum. Scientists suspect that aluminum accumulates in long-lived cells such as nerve cells, where it acts as a neurotoxin causing degenerative damage in the brain. Aluminum enters the body most commonly through diet, including baking soda, salt, vitamins, and even toothpaste. The main source of aluminum is industrial polluters, cooking utensils and appliances.

Nitrates. Nitrates result mostly from agricultural runoff and seepage from septic tanks. They enter both surface and well water and have caused "baby blue" syndrome (methemoglobinemia). In adults, they can help manufacture nitrosamines, which are known carcinogens. Boiling water increases nitrate concentration.

A quarter of all private wells in Iowa, Kansas, Minnesota, Nebraska and S. Dakota are contaminated by excessive levels of nitrate. In fact, nitrate contaminated water supplies have been found in practically every corn belt state.

Iron. Iron is a commonly available mineral that gives your water the unsavory orange-red color you usually see first thing in the morning. Although it certainly detracts from your water's aesthetic, it is not a dangerous metal. Its main damage is to the taste or color of your coffee or tea. Iron is actually a necessary mineral used in the manufacture of red blood cells. It is a transporter of oxygen and is needed to prevent anemia. Common filters will remove the rust.

Radioactivity. Radioactive pollution in drinking water is a serious problem. Atomic power plants, military weapons and new medical techniques create radioactive waste products and disposing of them is a problem. Leaks with measurable effects on aquatic life have appeared in the oceans where 20-30 years ago the first dumps were created. Part of the criteria for a nuclear dump is that it have the capacity to prevent leaks for over 10,000 years—the time it takes for radioactivity to decay to safe levels.

Much radiation contamination in this country stems from the effluent waters released by uranium mines and power plants in New Mexico, Colorado, Iowa, Illinois, Wisconsin, and Missouri. At present, no one has determined the long range effects of low level radiation and how much is tolerable in water. Even spring water can have radionuclides, since it passes through soil and rocks that may naturally radiate or be contaminated. Plutonium and radium contamination are causes of bone and liver cancer. Radiation affects fetuses and the newborn causing mutagenic cell division resulting in abnormal birth or development.

Radon. The EPA estimates 17 million Americans are threatened by excessive radon levels. Radon is a radioactive gas that permeates ground water in New Jersey, New England, and the Western Mountain States. Preliminary studies found that radon in drinking water can double the risk of soft tissue cancers.

Mercury. Prolonged ingestion of mercury can result in loss of muscle control, kidney disease, and brain damage. The National Wildlife Federation reported that snow and rain in the Midwest contains mercury levels in excess of EPA safe limits. Mercury levels were found to be 42 times EPA safe levels in Chicago and 65 times EPA safe levels in Detroit.[40]

In mercury contaminated rivers and lakes, mercury entered the brains of trout through nerves that connect water exposed sensory receptors. This is the first evidence that mercury crosses the blood-brain barrier, thought to be an almost impermeable membrane. The Canadian and Swedish scientists conducting this study concluded, extrapolating to humans, "that mercury and other toxins could accumulate in human brains via nerve transport."[41] This is especially true for children and fetuses.

Copper and PVC Piping

By current EPA standards, copper pipes are acceptable and copper tubing is used in many under-the-sink filters. But if blue or blue-green stains appear in the sink, it usually means that the copper plumbing fixtures are corroding. Aquarium fish die from copper contaminated water. Polyvinylchloride (PVC) pipes can leach vinyl chloride into the water causing damage to kidneys, the nervous system, the liver, the immune, and circulatory systems.

To Test or to Treat?

The United States has made tremendous advances in the last 25 years to clean up its waterways. But the job is so enormous that we still cannot expect to drink any water, fish in any river, or swim in any lake. Beach closures, fish kills, and oil spills still plague our headline news. Pure rain water falls from the sky and crystal clear snow melts from the highest mountain tops. But as they drip through our ecosystem, they pick up industrial wastes, agricultural chemicals, and micro-organisms. After that, there are the chemicals we add to our water intentionally in order to "purify" it.

Municipal water suppliers are required to mail annual water quality statements that list amounts of contaminants and tell whether government standards have been met. Unfortunately, these reports may be unintelligible to the average person. Even if you could understand it all, there are other problems. Those tests were done on water at the plant, so contaminants like lead, iron, mercury, and chlorine byproducts such as THMs will not be listed. Also chemical and pesticide contamination often fall within "acceptable" federal health standards because they are based on economic feasibility. Of the hundreds of pollutants in our water, only dozens are tested for. The cost of testing water for hundreds of contaminants can be as costly as a home filtration system that removes those pollutants.

To find out more about public drinking water safety standards, and where your local water comes from, contact the EPA's Safe Drinking Water Hotline, *800-426-4791* www.EPA.gov/safewater.

Which Water Is Right for You?

A Primer on Bottled Waters and Home Water Treatment Devices

The effects of water pollution are widespread and the dangers are obvious. Nevertheless, in our present political climate, even such important issues as these become mired in bureaucratic mud. Thus, the problem trickles down to one of individual responsibility. When it comes time to wet your palate, the decision of what to drink and what to avoid is yours alone. Perhaps this is the way it ought to be. If we don't make that decision, one day the government may make it for us. But herein also lies a burden—that of educating oneself about the numerous options. What follows is a discussion of many of those options for buying or making clean drinking, cooking, and bathing water.

Some Alternatives to Tap Water

a) Bottled Water
b) Charcoal/Carbon Filtered Water
c) Home Distilled Water
d) Ozone and Ultraviolet Treated Water
e) Reverse Osmosis Treated Water

For Most of Us, This Bubbles up a Lot of Questions

Is bottled water safe? Which one is best? What is a distiller? What makes the price of one water treatment device $20 and another over $1,000. How do I know which one I need?

This list of questions can get long and the decision so forbidding and technical that the easiest choice is to do nothing. Buying bottled water from the supermarket is often the result of this non-decision. After all, home water cleaning equipment requires an investment and unlike cars, you cannot take them for a test drive. Consumer magazines may on occasion compare bottled waters, filters, or distillers, but rarely do they contrast the different categories against each other. Yet, you the consumer, require this kind of information to make an educated decision that is correct for your health, pocketbook, and lifestyle.

One caveat about our discussion of the different waters. Perfection is unattainable. While these waters do their job of reducing certain contaminants to healthy levels, it is incorrect to assume that any bottled water or water treatment device removes 100% of everything or anything. True, in many cases, we can achieve 99% and even 99.9% reduction of a contaminant. But filters age and conditions change and what was once 99% may now be less. Suffice it to say that when you see such terms as "eliminates" or "removes" or "purifies," while they may be true overall, you cannot assume them to indicate 100% perfection. "Pure" and "clean" are unattainable ideals. However, as you read on, you will definitely find there are numerous ways to get safe, healthy, and delicious water for you and your family.

Bottled, Spring, and Mineral Waters

Cool down and have a drink of bottled water. No matter where you go, from rural roadside gas stations to ethnic groceries, gourmet stores, and supermarkets here and around the world, you will find numerous brands of bottled water. Bottled water in the USA alone is a $4 billion industry, with consumption growing at a rate of 45% from 1992 to 1997. In 1976 Americans drank 1.5 gallons of bottled water per person. In 1999, they drank 17 gallons per person making bottled water the fastest growing beverage in the country and more popular than fruit drinks.

Americans are still just novices when compared to Europeans who have known about the benefits of bottled water for years. "Mineral" water is the term used for water that is rich in "beneficial" minerals. It usually comes from deep underground springs or artesian wells and contains at least 250 parts per million of dissolved solids—usually calcium, magnesium, sodium, potassium, silica, and bicarbonates. Some minerals, such as sulfur, have given health spas their reputation for amazing cures. Is it any wonder? Many of our medicines are sulfa drugs. Some foreign sources of mineral water bottled at their source include:

Perrier	France
S. Pellegrino	Italy
Apollinaris	Germany
Vichy	France
Fiuggi	Italy
Evian	France
Volvic	France

Some American bottled water brands of are:

Trinity	Diamond Natural
Saratoga Vichy	Great Bear
Mountain Valley	Dasani
Arrowhead Mountain Spring	Aquafina
Poland Spring	Deer Park
Zephyrhills	Crystal Springs
Le Bleu	Le Glacéau

Once considered to be a convenience service industry providing water coolers for offices, schools and public buildings, bottled water is now sold in pints and quart bottles and considered a gourmet item by some, while others consider it a necessity. But where does bottled water come from? It can trickle down from mountains or spring up from deep artesian wells. Spring water comes from the earth flowing naturally from an underground spring. Some spring water is naturally carbonated, others have added carbon dioxide to make the bubbles. Mineral waters are spring waters with high counts of mineral salts that are renowned for their ancient healing qualities. They can also be naturally carbonated, or improved with added carbon dioxide gas. Some bottled drinking waters are municipal waters that have been cleaned up through filtration and/or ozonation. Unlike regular tap water, this water is purer and has never traveled through miles of aging underground pipes. By and large, bottled waters are a boon to our health and safety, but they are not without their problems.

Problems with Bottled Waters

In 1998, the National Resources Defense Council completed a 4 year test of 103 bottled waters and found that one-third of them contained bacteria and other chemicals exceeding industry standards. It showed deficiencies in industry regulation. That is likely because 43 of the 50 US states have the equivalent of fewer than one single staff person dedicated to regulating bottled water. Some states have no regulations at all for bottled water. In an early pilot survey on bottled water, the Environmental Protection Agency found that the actual chemical composition of the water did not always match the label information, and trace amounts of chlorine, nitrates, copper, manganese, lead, iron, zinc, mercury, and/or arsenic were found. Chemical and bacteriological analysis were not performed regularly, and when they were, there were quality control problems such as incomplete chemical analyses for the source water or the processed (bottled) water.

The newest problem is bottled water tampering. In September of 2000, New York City was plagued with a series of incidents involving bottled water scares when two dozen people complained of mouth burns after drinking from bottles of Perrier, Aquafina, and Poland Spring. Health officials said the waters were contaminated with ammonia, sodium hydroxide, and chlorine.

Some bottlers treat their water with ozone, deionization, carbon and micron filtration, and ultraviolet light to purify it. Perrier, for example, uses ozonation to treat their bottled water in several of their American plants. Perrier's bottled water brands include Arrowhead Mountain Spring Water, Perrier, and Zephyrhills.

Mineral waters may also be high in minerals like sodium, arsenic, or cobalt. When Consumer Reports Magazine tested bottled waters in the summer of 2000, it found several brands above the EPA's proposed standard for arsenic. Previous investigations have found sodium counts as high as a whopping 397 milligrams.[42] (People on low-sodium diets should avoid water with high sodium content.) In September, 2000, employees of a software company in Albany, NY became violently ill after drinking from their water cooler supplied by the Diamond Springs Water Co. of Troy, NY. Analysis found that the 5-gallon bottle contained a petroleum product similar to gasoline. Diamond Springs' source is spring water which is subjected to ultraviolet light and a one micron filtration process to screen out giardia and cryptosporidium.

FDA regulations require bottled water be processed, packaged, transported, and stored under safe and sanitary conditions. Bottlers must monitor their source waters and their finished products for contaminants.

The *International Bottled Water Association*, the industry trade group, sets strict inspection standards covering everything from sanitation rules for employees and filling room equipment, to annual chemical and physical tests including possible unannounced inspections.

One of the oldest and best known American mineral waters is Mountain Valley, which is forced up through a bed of marble in the remote valley of Hot Springs, Arkansas. In 1832, President Andrew Jackson commissioned a study of the water that eventually led to the protection of dozens of thermal springs around the U.S. So deep is Hot Springs, that chemical assays of its mineral content have remained virtually unchanged for the last 60 years.

The world's deepest known source for bottled spring water is Trinity Springs in Paradise, Idaho, adjacent to the Sawtooth National Forest. The spring is 2.2 miles deep; that is equivalent to standing eight Empire State buildings on top of each other. Trinity's geothermal water forces its way up through faults in this mass and reaches the surface at a seething 138°F. A batholith of solid granite carbon-dated at 16,000 years protects the water from contamination by other groundwaters.

Happily, the people at Trinity are committed to not altering the water from its organic state in any way. It is neither pasteurized nor ozonated, but bottled in the traditional European way, without processing. This water has been classified as a mineral dietary supplement under the Dietary Supplement Health and Education Act (DSHEA) because of its silica content.

Non-Source Bottled Water

According to the *International Bottled Water Association* (IBWA), there is a one in four chance that your bottled water has been drawn from municipal taps. America's best selling bottled water is Aquafina, which is treated tap water packaged by Pepsi. Not to be outdone, Coke makes the popular water Dasani. Even New York City is bottling its water and selling it throughout New York State with the motto: "Forget the rest, drink the best." These are called"non-source" waters because they do not arise from a spring, artesian well, or other natural source. In fact, they can come from anywhere. Aquafina, for example, originates from 16 not-very-exotic sources such as Detroit, Fresno, and Munster, Indiana. Typically, they are treated with ozone, de-ionization, carbon and micron filtration, and ultraviolet light to improve their quality and keep them safe. Essentia water of Woodinville, Washington has huge reverse osmosis machines to clean up their water as does Aquafina and Dasani. Le Bleu Ultra Pure of Winston Salem, North Carolina, and Nascar Premium steam distill their waters as does Le Glacéau (Energy brands). These non-source bottled waters can be safer and cleaner than natural waters. Choose the treatment method you trust most, when purchasing non-source bottled waters.

Plastic Bottles and Storage Containers

Some bottlers, such as Mountain Valley, Perrier, and S. Pellegrino, use glass. Unfortunately, glass costs 1-2 times more than plastic and is heavy and breakable. Plastic bottles thus dominate the marketplace.

Some kinds of plastic can impart a plastic taste to water. This means it is imparting plastic. This is a frustrating irony considering the reason you purchase bottled water in the first place is to avoid pollutants. Water bottled in PETE (or PET–polyethylene tereph-thalate), a clear, strong plastic, is considered the most inert. Look for #1 in the triangle on the bottom of the bottle. Some PETE bottles are firmer than others, meaning the bottler uses thicker plastic for a more durable product. Gallon and 4 liter jugs are often bottled in high-density polyethylene (HDPE), a flaccid, opaque plastic bottle, that has the greatest potential to impart a plastic taste. It has #2 in the triangle on the bottom of the bottle. Polyvinyl chloride, PVC, is much sturdier and less likely to impart taste, but is not as widely used. It has #3 in the triangle on the bottom of the bottle. Polycarbonate plastic is strong and rigid and is the kind most often used for 5-gallon water cooler jugs. It is highly inert, and imparts no taste and has been used for water bottles, baby bottles, and food storage containers for 35 years. Look for #7 in the triangle on the bottom of the bottle.

Convenience and Availability

Logistics is another consideration when using bottled water. For example, what would you do if your bottle ran dry and it was 11 p.m. on a snowy mid-winter night? Would you hop over to the grocery in your pajamas, fighting the cold, snow, and ice? Most of us would simply drink from the tap and rationalize: "....a little bit is okay..." But the risk of drinking any amount of contaminated water is not worth it. Getting clean water should not involve questions of convenience. And that includes weight: Imagine lugging in a bundle of groceries and a couple of jugs of water up the stairs! If you drink bottled water, consider paying a little extra for delivery service.

The availability of pure water ought not to involve consider-ations of price. The average household uses between 2½ to 3 gallons of water each day for drinking and cooking purposes. That adds up to about 1,000 gallons or, about $1,000 dollars per year. That is quite a sum for something that should be free in the first place! This does not even include usage for such things as watering

your plants, feeding your pets, growing sprouts, etc. But it should!
Plants and animals like people, prefer non-chlorinated water.

Read The Label

Another problem with bottled water is fraud. Many waters
represented as "spring" or "spring fresh" water, are in fact filtered
municipal water. Some companies legally slip this by the consumer
with clever labeling. One label has "spring" in the name of the
brand, for example "Paterson SPRING Water Co." Since the word
"spring" is the largest word on the label, consumers take it for
granted that it is spring water. The logo for Great Bear bottled
water from Breinigsville, PA is a polar bear on ice, but it is not
glacier water.

Fortunately, the *International Bottled Water Association
(IBWA)*, sets standards about purity and labeling for its members.
But assuming that bottlers are true to their advertising may be
asking a lot. Brand trustworthiness has been challenged in the
highly competitive climate of the marketplace. Your decision is
tough. Should you spend more money for a"name brand" or is
"brand X" just as good? The answer requires a little detective
work.

Understanding a Chemical Assay

Don't worry, you won't need your Sherlock Holmes pipe, just
a paper and pen. Start by writing each company and requesting the
chemical analysis or "assay," of their water. You will receive a list
of their water's ingredients that should look something like this:

Pollutant	Deer Park Water	Poland Spring[43]
Nitrates	.21mg/l	.15mg/l
Fluoride	.100	.100
Organic Halides	.007	.004
Chloride	5.700	3.100
Iron	.030	.030
Sodium	2.000	3.000
Hardness	17.000	32.500
Aluminum	.135	.100

Other elements listed in the assay may be:

Bacteria	Color
Turbidity	Odor
Lead	Foaming Agents
Arsenic	TDS
Mercury	Coliform bacteria
pH (acidity)	Sodium
Sulfates	Phosphates

Organic halides refer to the pollutants that form THMs (trihalomethanes). Turbidity is the cloudiness of water. TDS means the total amount of dissolved solids. You may also find common pesticides. Interpreting the significance of these statistics is the hard job. After all your statistics arrive, compare the different waters. Is .135 aluminum a dangerous amount? Is .007 halides too much? How much arsenic is okay? The real question becomes: Do I know enough to evaluate these reports? Do I have the time and ambition to learn more about this aspect of water quality?

Some Criteria for Choosing Quality Bottled Water

☞ Choose a water that has stable assay statistics over years.
☞ Arrange for home delivery. Convenience means consistency.
☞ Buy water in glass, polycarbonate, or PETE bottles.
☞ Choose quality over price.
☞ Know the difference between spring, mineral, and purified waters and make the choice that suits you best.

Unfortunately, for most of us, the comparison of chemical assays waters down to a soggy headache. For many, the choice among bottled waters boils down to an unscientific "eeny-meeny-miny-mo." Is this how you want to pick your drinking water? Even if you were knowledgeable enough to evaluate the reports, there are other questions such as: how recent is the assay report? Are these statistics consistent? Or do they vary month-to-month? Does the analysis list the particular pollutants about which you are most concerned? Are offensive results being edited out? Another big question is: who did the test? Does the water company use a reputable, certified, independent lab? Do they alternate labs to corroborate findings?

Not all bottled waters are equal! High quality bottled water does indeed exist. But we consumers must make the effort to find them. After all, buying bottled water for drinking and cooking represents a considerable annual investment. And this is surely one case where we are putting our money where our mouth is!

Charcoal Water Filters

The term "filters" refers to a class of water cleaning devices that have one basic thing in common—charcoal. It is simply carbon ash, but it has been treating drinking water since biblical times. Charcoal has no superior when it comes to the adsorption of organic compounds, gases, odors, and tastes. Pharmacists and nature-doctors still use it today for complaints of intestinal gas. Hospitals use it in kidney dialysis machines. Pet owners use it in fish tanks and industries use it in everything from gas masks to cigarette filters.

Granular Activated Carbon Filters

"Activated" carbon refers to charcoal that has been exposed to high temperatures and steam in the absence of oxygen. Vegetable charcoal, often derived from coconut hulls, is the most common material used. The result of activation is a honeycomb-like super-structure that is filled with millions of tiny tunnels. This granular activated carbon (GAC) contains a microscopic labyrinth with an enormous surface area on which carbon molecules can cling. This is the reason for carbon's fantastic adsorptive capacity. One pound of granular activated carbon provides a surface area equivalent to 125 acres!

Simple charcoal filters for treating tap water are widely available in department, kitchen, and housewares stores and even supermarkets. They range in price from $20 to $60. More sophisticated charcoal filters can cost in the $200 to $400 range. The wide span of prices reflects major differences in quantity of charcoal, design, durability, convenience, and most importantly, scope of pollutants treated. But the real cost of a filter is found in the expense of its replacement cartridges. These are like razor blades to the razor. Before you buy, check the cost of replacements. You will be replacing the filter cartridges as little as once per year to as much as twelve times per year and it will be your primary expense. If a cartridge costs $75 and lasts for 500 gallons, for example, your water cost is 15¢ per gallon.

On the low end of charcoal filters is the common carafe filter. Basically, this is a water pitcher that filters like a coffee maker. Tap water is poured into the top, runs down through a small filter, and the filtered water lands at the bottom. It significantly reduces chlorine, gases, odors, and tastes. The carafe is inexpensive (approximately $20), portable, and easy to use. But, the filters need to be changed one to two times per month to avoid bacterial growth. Based on the cost of a typical replacement filter, this amounts to approximately 30 cents per gallon. This frequent changing is also bothersome for most folks who slack off on their filter-changing responsibilities. This laziness can result in water that is more contaminated than what comes out of the tap!

Faucet mounted canisters are another inexpensive ($25-$60) type of charcoal filter. They contain small amounts of charcoal. In some brands, tap water may drill a hole through the center of the canister because the charcoal is loosely packed. This makes for a speedy flow rate but minimal contact time with the charcoal. These filters also need to be changed frequently to avoid bacterial growth. Their charcoal can also be damaged by the unintentional usage of hot water. High end faucet mounted filters may include micron strainers to effectively remove cysts such as giardia and cryptosporidium. Some even have bypasses for hot water and monitors to remind you to change the filter. They can remove chlorine, gases, odors, tastes and reduce volatile organic compounds (VOCs), trihalomethanes (THMs), and pesticides.

All simple charcoal filters should be replaced frequently. Dark, moist charcoal turns out to be an ideal breeding ground for bacteria. After a few weeks, the bacterial population is large enough to leak out of the filter. Old filters can only hold so much. Some units actually start to unload their pollutants when they reach their saturation point, recontaminating the water.[44]

A better carbon filter is the tall column model. These range from 6 inches to 2 feet and contain large quantities of densely packed charcoal. The water moves down the long tube, getting cleaner and cleaner as it journeys to the bottom. These units can be installed at the point where the water enters the house, or under a sink, or on the countertop. Countertop units connect to the faucet via a tube and often have a spigot at their top to dispense the filtered water. They range in price from $50-$200 and effectively remove chlorine, gases, odors, tastes and reduce an even greater percentage of volatile organic compounds (VOCs), trihalomethanes (THMs), and pesticides.

Carbon Block Filters

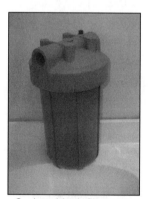

Carbon block filters are so densely packed that if flattened out they would cover the surface of a tennis court.

So far the carbon filters we have discussed do an excellent job of reducing two categories of pollutants: aesthetic impurities such as those that affect water taste, odor, and turbidity; and health impurities such as pesticides, VOCs, THMs, gases, and many other organic compounds. Carbon block filters begin to work in a third area, that of inorganics, metals, and bacteria.

Carbon block filters contain great volumes of charcoal compressed into super-dense blocks. Most also include layers of other media that filter the water before and after the charcoal. The technology behind carbon blocks can get very sophisticated. Some use different activating processes that create new geometric lattices that increase the adsorptive area. They range in price from $200-$400. They effectively remove chlorine, toxic gases, odors, tastes, VOCs, THMs, pesticides, organic compounds, heavy metals such as lead, and bacteria and cysts such as E. coli, protozoa, giardia, and cryptosporidium.

These units are often mounted under the sink where they connect directly to the cold water pipe. On the sinktop, all you see is a fountain spigot. Countertop models use the same filter cartridge but have a housing that attaches to the faucet end via a double tube. The faucet works normally for washing dishes but when a valve is pressed, water travels to and through the filter in one tube and returns to the faucet via the second tube. These countertop models install easily. Just screw the included diverter valve onto the faucet tip. The undersink models require tapping into the cold water line and possibly drilling a hole for the new filter spigot. This may require a plumber. Both models last from 400 to 1,000 gallons which results in your replacing the filter one to three times per year.

When shopping for this kind of filter, consider flow rate. Some filters are so densely packed, it can get rather tedious waiting for a glass of water. However, this is preferred to the kind that "gushes" forth. Filters with slow flow rates of under one half gallon per minute, generally provide good quality water by increasing the contact time of the water and charcoal. Flow rate also depends, of course, on your water pressure.

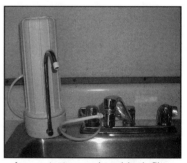

A countertop carbon block filter with its own pure water spigot. A diverter valve on the faucet end switches between tap water and filtered water.

Charcoal filters are most effective early in their life and decrease their efficiency as the carbon's available surface area is filled up. Thus, if you have very dirty water with lots of large particle matter, it will make sense to use a pre-filter so that the adsorptive capacity of the carbon is not wasted on fibers, rust, dirt, etc. In better models, you will know when to change the filter because they have monitors that signal you by checking for decreasing flow rate.

Pros and Cons of Charcoal Filters

(See chart) Bacteria is probably the greatest problem with basic charcoal filters because they can actually promote the propagation of bacteria, yeasts, molds, cysts, and other micro-organisms. Microorganisms love the dark, wet environment of a filter. The chlorine in your tap cannot get rid of all bacteria; it only keeps their counts low. Once your filter removes the chlorine, the bacteria multiply and feed off the trapped organic pollutants in it. This is a major disadvantage of charcoal filters. If you do not change the filter, you run the risk of breeding more bacteria than was in the original water!

The big question is then, how do you know when to change the filter? Most manufacturers will recommend a change period. But there are other variables such as your rate of usage or the age of your plumbing. Bacteria may build up to harmful levels in as little as 2–3 weeks. But how would you know? After all, bacteria don't come out and whistle!

What to Look for When Buying a Charcoal Filter

- Large amounts of densely packed charcoal
- Long filter life, preferably 400-1000 gallons
- Pre-filter to prolong the main filter's life
- Maximum contact time and reasonable flow rate
- Countertop unit connects directly to the faucet
- Under the sink unit saves space and is out of sight
- Hard side walls to maintain the integrity of the solid carbon block and prevent breakdown or contaminant feedback

---

Pros & Cons of Charcoal Filtration

Advantages

- Best method for extracting toxic gases, odors, and tastes
- Best method for extracting all organic, hydrocarbon based pollutants such as pesticides, chlorine, THMs, and PCBs
- Most economical filtration method
- Some models have ability to reduce heavy metals such as lead, cadmium, and chromium
- Some carbon block models can prevent entry of bacteria and pathogens such as giardia & E. coli

Disadvantages

- Does not remove inorganic mineral salts such as sodium, fluoride, and nitrates
- Has little affect on soluble minerals, or asbestos fibers
- Provides a breeding ground for bacteria
- Has a limited life
- Difficult to determine when filter's effectiveness is used up
- Destroyed by hot water
- Carbon in some filters can break down and return contaminants to the drinking water

How do you know when to change your filter? Look for: a change in taste, odor, or color; a reduction in the flow rate; or the appearance of cloudiness or small particles. More sophisticated charcoal filters include monitors that signal you when they register a slower flow rate, indicating an aging filter, and others contain micro-strainers that prevent bacteria from exiting or entering the unit.

Another problem for charcoal is stagnation. If you use a filter for one week, and go on vacation the second week, you will likely return to a house with a million guests—bacteria! Manufacturers generally do not warn you about bacteria, for fear of scaring their audience. Nor would it be good business to suggest that you change your filters every couple of weeks. Others neglect to tell you *not* to use hot water. The adsorptive properties of charcoal are damaged by hot water and worse, it may liberate the contaminants held within.

Submicron-Straining Carbon Purifiers

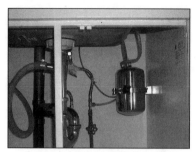

An undersink installation of a submicron carbon block filter.

Some high-end carbon block filters are designed with submicron-strainers that wrap around the carbon core and prevent bacteria from either entering or leaving the filter cartridge. These units physically strain out ninety-nine percent of bacteria. Bacteria are generally larger than one micron in size, but micro-straining carbon filters can strain down to half that size, 0.5 microns, or better. To give you an idea of just how small this is, a human hair is 100 microns thick and a red blood cell is 0.9 microns! This effectively eliminates cysts like cryptosporidium and giardia, pathogenic bacteria such as E. coli, salmonella, fungi, yeasts, and parasites, as well as tiny asbestos fibers that pass through ordinary carbon filters.

Bacteria are either prevented from entering the media or are trapped and never make it out. The technology for this kind of superfine straining was developed for the Gemini Space Program so astronauts could purify their own water in space. However, micro-straining carbon block filters do not remove viruses, which are 20 to 100 times smaller than bacteria. Nor do they eliminate inorganic chemicals, salts, or ions like fluoride, nitrates, and sodium. Only distillation and reverse osmosis methods can reduce these.

Some of these carbon block strainers enhance their filtration with other technologies such as electrostatically charged layers. This could be a blend of cotton or cellulose that has been given a positive molecular charge. Since most colloidal pollutants, bacteria, and inorganic compounds exhibit a negative charge in solution, this filter layer absorbs the charged particles by electrokinetic attraction. The effect is similar to the way lint is attracted to wool.

This provides reduction of some contaminants that are not picked up by micro-straining. The materials used in these purifiers are insoluble and chemically inactive themselves. They work by exerting a catalytic effect, inducing molecular changes in many chemicals contained within the water. It is for this reason that some of these devices can extract a small percentage of negatively charged fluoride ions and even some dissolved minerals.

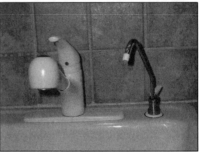

With an undersink installation, all you can see on your counter is a spigot

All these devices have their limits and their capacity to reduce contaminants deteriorates over time. Advertising claims about endurance can be misleading. Everyone's water is different and different conditions affect the life and performance of your filter. A conscientious manufacturer should test his unit at the maximum age limit of the device. In any event, it behooves you, as a lay person, to change your filter regularly and at the first suspicion of deterioration. One marker is a change in odor and taste. Although the filter may still be effective for other contaminants, these two changes are easy to detect and are indications of an aging filter. As an alternative, simply mark your calendar with filter-change dates and stick to it.

Pros and Cons of Micro-Straining Carbon Filters

The major advantage of a good micro-straining carbon block filter is the convenient elimination of bacteria. These devices provide water on demand, use no electricity, have easy maintenance, and easy installation. They waste no water, and effectively remove a wide range of pollutants including microscopic size microorganisms. With all these features and affordable prices, they make a superb choice for many homes. You turn the knob and you get water. Isn't that the way it should be?

Disadvantages: hard carbon block micro-strainers still cannot remove inorganic minerals such as fluoride, nitrates, sulfates, sodium, and sub-micron size organisms such as viruses.

Ceramic Filters

Ceramic filters are made from diatomaceous earth, volcanic sand, or magnetite stone. They've been around since 1835 when Queen Victoria of England commissioned Henry Doulton to purify and protect the royal drinking water from the cholera epidemic in London. Doulton filters still exist today. They eliminate any worries about cholera, dysentery, giardia, cysts, e-coli, or cryptosporidium. The microscopic pores inside the ceramic trap bacteria as small as 0.2-0.5 microns, which is considered bacteriologically sterile. Ceramic filters are also very economical, lasting for 2,000-3,000 gallons. And they are washable—just scrub them with a brush under cold water. But like other systems, ceramics need to be supplemented to cover a full range of pollutants. By itself, it cannot remove viruses, dissolved solids, or inorganic salts such as fluorides, nitrates, and heavy metals. Typically, ceramics are combined with charcoal, activated alumina, and/or silver. The charcoal eliminates organic chemicals, chlorine, bad taste, and odor. The alumina absorbs fluoride, and the silver kills the trapped bacteria so they cannot regrow. Prices range from $200–$400.

KDF and Shower Filters

While the purity of our drinking water is of primary importance, contaminants such as chlorine and its byproducts also enter our bodies through the skin. Our lungs also absorb toxic fumes from the gaseous chlorine byproducts that are released in a steamy shower. A report in *Science News* estimated we inhale enough pollutants in a ten minute shower to equal drinking a gallon of polluted water. Chlorine in shower water can strip protein from our

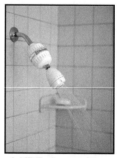

A KDF shower filter.

hair and skin causing dry, irritated eyes, itchy skin, and dandruff. Hair can become dull and carry a chlorine smell. This is why people need to wear swimming caps! Filtering shower water also helps control bacteria and fight bathroom mold and mildew.

Shower filters attach directly to the showerhead or replace the showerhead itself. While charcoal is supremely effective for removing chlorine, the volume of water used in a shower is so large that the frequency of refills would make it uneconomical. A new ion binding medium, known as KDF significantly reduces chlorine and heavy metals, and has a much longer life.

Advantages of KDF Filtration

- **Eliminates Chlorine:** Converts free chlorine to harmless chloride
- **Reduces Heavy Metals:** Redox principle changes lead ions in water to lead atoms which electroplate onto KDF surface
- **Reduces Scale:** Alters the nature of limescale, changes crystalline structure so that scale turns into powder
- **Kills Bacteria:** KDF possesses inherent toxicity to bacteria

---

KDF is a patented copper-zinc alloy that filters by a process called reduction oxidation. Here is how it works. Since water is neutral, neither positively nor negatively charged, any particle that has a charge will be attracted to the filter. Pollutants actually bond to the zinc and copper. When a charged particle loses or gains electrons, it changes its composition. This changeover is known as reduction oxidation or redox for short.

Through this redox process, potentially harmful chemicals become harmless. Zinc reduces chlorine to soluble zinc chloride. Copper reacts with hydrogen sulfide to form cupric sulfide and scale changes from glass to powder. KDF is also effective in reducing lead, iron, arsenic, mercury, and hydrogen sulfide. After water has been in contact with KDF, oxygen-depleting bacteria cannot grow. And unlike charcoal, KDF functions in both hot and cold water conditions without deterioration. Range $40-$80.

Most shower filters can also be backwashed to optimize their performance. Life of a good KDF filter is above 10,000 gallons, far superior to charcoal and about a years worth of showers and baths. KDF filters generally range in price from $50-$125. When buying a shower filter, check the ease of removal, installation, and reversal for backwashing.

Water Softeners

Water softeners are not filters. They do not clean the water, but rather change its behavior. Precipitated calcium and magnesium in water leave a film of sediment on hair, clothing, pipes, dishes, bathtubs, and prevent soap from lathering. Soft water exists naturally, but if the water in your area is naturally hard, you can treat it with a water softener. Conventional water softeners add salt to water in a process of ion exchange that reduces the high calcium and magnesium content, but can also elevate sodium levels in your drinking water. Magnetic water softeners operate by breaking up the large calcium carbonate molecules with their magnetic polarization. The calcium then dissolves and the suds return to your soap.

Bactericides

A bactericide is an agent that can render water safe from harmful bacteria and other microorganisms including parasites, amoebae, protozoa, algae, cysts, and viruses that have a long history of causing waterborne diseases such as typhoid, dysentery, and hepatitis, among others. This is sharply distinct from simple charcoal water filters that, as we have seen, are incapable of such a task. The most common bactericides in use are the chemicals chlorine, bromine, iodine, and silver, along with ultraviolet light, and ozone gas.

Chlorine

By now, it is public knowledge that chlorine, added to the water supply to kill bacteria, combines with other chemicals to create a host of cancer causing by-products. But what is not so well known is that this famous bactericide is not so dependable against larger organisms such as cysts, amoebae, protozoa, and others. This first came to light in the late 1970s when the *National Academy of Sciences* reported 99 outbreaks of waterborne diseases in the U.S. including an epidemic of giardia cysts found in chlorinated water!

Bromine

Bromine is a well-known germicide, but because of its high cost it is almost never used in public water supplies. Its most common application is in industry and as a swimming pool disinfectant. It is quite effective against microorganisms, even more so than chlorine and does not cause "swimmers red eye" and other common chlorine side effects.

Iodine

Iodine is capable of destroying cysts, bacteria, and viruses, and is most popular with campers, travelers, and the military. Iodine, in itself, is a nutrient, but iodinated organic compounds may be formed in water with potential toxicity. For this reason it is not recommended for long term use or by pregnant mothers.

Silver

Silver has been used as a bactericide for a long time, but it has fallen from popularity. One of the main difficulties in using it for water purification is that it requires a long retention time. Silver is a slow working bactericide that has to stay in contact with the water for a fairly long time.

Iodine, bromine, and chlorine, although stronger than silver, also require adequate dosage and time to get the job done. Various factors may actually increase the amount of time necessary. With chlorine, for example, a tiny amount of ammonia in the water (from agricultural runoff or decaying leaves) can increase the amount of holding time required. Other common elements such as iron and sulfur also "use up" the chlorine, bromine, iodine, or silver, making them unavailable for killing bacteria. With typical water flow rates of up to one gallon per minute, this may not be sufficient time for the silver in the filter to do its job. In addition, with all these chemical bactericides, the combination of silver and other chemicals in the water may form potentially toxic compounds, not to mention the unsavory thought of drinking water that includes dead bacteria.

Ultraviolet Light

The same type of germicidal lamp used in hospitals and laboratories can be used to kill germs in water. These lamps produce short wave beams of (light) radiation that are lethal to bacteria, viruses and other microorganisms. Water enters the ultraviolet (UV) purifier and flows into the ring between the bulb and the stainless steel outside chamber wall. It takes only seconds to destroy most microorganisms.

These special lamps use about 10-60 watts of electricity and can last as long as 7,500 hours. Thousands of gallons of water can be treated for an extremely low operating cost. And the appliances are low maintenance. Ultraviolet devices have great potential, but they do need supplementation with charcoal or ceramics. One caveat to watch for, is that they share the same dilemma of contact time vs. effectiveness as charcoal and chlorine. The longer the exposure to UV light, the more effective. A one-half gallon per minute flow rate, for example, allows enough UV exposure to kill the resilient cryptosporidium eggs. A faster flowing UV unit may not provide enough exposure to sterilize the water.

Ozone

Ozone is not new as a treatment for water, nor is it unnatural. It was discovered in the late 18th century by a Dutch scientist who named it after the Greek word meaning "smell." Its smell is the pure smell of activated oxygen. Ozone is formed when oxygen (0_2) is agitated and split. The freed molecules of oxygen (0_1) temporarily jump on the backs of the regular oxygen forming 0_3. This condition lasts only for a few minutes as the 0_3 form of oxygen is unstable and quickly returns to the normal 0_2. Ozone, or "active oxygen," is produced by lightening, or passing air through an electric field, or over the light from a particular wavelength (230 angstroms) in the ultraviolet range. The latter simulates the way nature makes ozone from sunlight.

Actually, we have been living with ozone all our lives and would be quite sick without it. Plants produce ozone on the tips of their leaves, which quickly turns into the oxygen they so generously provide us. Mountain top communities are known for their good health and longevity due, perhaps in part, to the higher ozone levels in the air. The "Ozone Layer," located in the upper levels of the atmosphere, protects us from harmful ultraviolet radiation emanating from the sun. This natural shield is being eaten away by fluorocarbon emissions from industry, air conditioners, and refrigerators. This is the same problem that forced the elimination of aerosol cans in the 1970s. Because of our diminishing ozone layer, ultraviolet rays are penetrating the atmosphere to a greater extent than ever before and are multiplying the incidence of skin cancer in overindulgent sunbathers.

Ozone is one of our most powerful natural germicides. In a study entitled *"A comparison of the bactericidal activity of ozone and chlorine,"* ozone was found to kill E. coli bacteria in less than one minute while chlorine took 1-10 minutes to have the same effect.[45] Other tests showed that ozone forms oxidizing agents in water that destroy pathogenic organisms such as cysts, viruses, amoebae, and spores, many of which are resistant to chlorine.[46] Ozone also sterilizes raw sewage containing a wide variety of toxins including botulism.[47] In a study done in 1969 entitled *"Ozone Treatment of Secondary Effluents from Wastewater Treatment Plants,"* ozone was determined to meet all U.S. requirements for chemical and bacteriologically safe water. Ozone turned toxic wastewater into drinking water with no color, odor, turbidity, or living organisms.[48]

Ozone works in two ways: oxidation and flocculation. Oxidation refers literally to the combustion of pollutants such as microorganisms, THMs, pesticides, chlorine, dioxin, etc. by adding an oxygen molecule to them. Flocculation refers to the transformation of insoluble salts—sodium, fluoride, nitrates, etc.—into larger soluble compounds that can then be filtered. Radioactive minerals, asbestos, and heavy metals are also reduced in this way.

Many countries use ozone for municipal water purification including Germany, Italy, France, and Canada. In the USA, Los Angeles has a large municipal ozone system and used it instead of chlorine for the swimming pools in their 1984 Olympics. Numerous other U.S. cities are using ozone as part of their water purification and it is popular with bottled water companies.

The Advantages of Ozone Are
• Destroys hard to kill pathogenic organisms
• Removes odors, tastes, and colors
• Oxidizes THMs, chlorine, pesticides
• Precipitates heavy metals, asbestos, fluoride, nitrates
• Actually helps aquatic life because it reverts back to oxygen
• Has potential for medical applications and air purification

In Comparison with Chlorine, Ozone Does Not
• Irritate the eyes, skin, or mucous membranes.
• Produce hazardous byproducts like THMs.
• Have corrosive side effects.

Isn't Ozone a Poison?

Unfortunately, there is a great deal of misunderstanding about this beneficial form of oxygen. The official government position is that ozone is a toxic gas; but in fact, it is quite harmless. As with most things, improper use can bring undesired results. Overzealous users of ozone air purifiers can irritate the mucous membranes of their nasal passages by breathing too much ozone. It drys out the membranes; but, so will too much oxygen. That is why oxygen is only 21% of our air. Ozone has another potential problem in that it can combine with nitrogen in the air (60% of our air is nitrogen) to form nitrous oxide. This is "laughing gas," the once popular anesthetic used by dentists. In any event, this effect does not occur in water purification, and ozone quantity can be easily adjusted in most air purifiers.

So, Where is It?

You have to search hard to find ozone water purifiers and part of the reason is economics. In swimming pools, ozone purification is about ten times more expensive than chlorination. As for municipal treatment plants, the research, development, retooling, installation, and financing costs, along with the politics, make it slow going. Home machines for air purification have become quite popular. Ozone for water purification, however, is still hard to find and at $400, is somewhat costly. When combined with a high density carbon prefilter, however, ozone offers a great deal of promise for home water purification.

Reverse Osmosis

Reverse osmosis is a mechanical process by which water gradually diffuses through a semipermeable membrane that refuses to allow the passage of certain contaminants. A typical reverse osmosis (RO) unit, attaches to your faucet which delivers water to the membrane. In normal osmosis, two solutions of different concentrations exist separated by the membrane. The water moves from the lesser concentrated solution in the direction of the

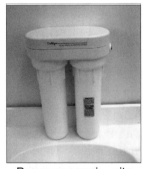

Reverse osmosis units are always combined with a carbon block filter.

greater concentration. In reverse osmosis, the more concentrated polluted water is forced under pressure in the direction of the pure water. Only the smallest molecules can penetrate the microscopic pores of the membrane. Most contaminants are left behind.

The great advantage of this type of filtration is its ability to significantly reduce pollutants in most major categories and operate without electricity. RO units provide one of the best methods of extracting inorganic minerals, heavy metals, lead, copper, cadmium, arsenic, and salts such as sulfates, nitrates, and fluoride. It also removes asbestos and, with the support of charcoal, virtually all organic chemicals and most aesthetic contaminants such as taste,

Reverse Osmosis

Effectively Removes	*Cannot Completely Remove*
Organic chemicals	Toxic Gases
Dissolved minerals	Chloroform
Nitrates, fluoride, sodium,	Phenol, THMs
sulfides, Cryptosporidium,	Some Pesticides
Giardia. Heavy metals,	Organic compounds of
lead, arsenic, radium.	low molecular weights
Asbestos, taste, odor.	Can grow bacteria

Pros	*Cons*
Uses no electricity	Uses 4-6 gallons of water to make
	one gallon of purified water.
Extracts most pollutants	Membrane replacement is costly.
including particulate	Requires pre & post carbon filters.
matter, lead, mercury,	Plumber installation required.
radium, uranium,	Water quality diminishes as
bacteria, viruses.	membrane ages.

odor, and color. The low mineral content (TDS) of RO treated water means it is suitable for steam irons, car batteries, and humidifiers. They accomplish all this with only water under pressure to operate.

The Center for Disease Control and Prevention (CDC) recommends reverse osmosis for preventing cryptosporidium and giardia contamination. The pore size of the RO membrane is smaller than these parasites, and also smaller than bacteria and viruses. However, even though bacteria cannot pass through the membrane, they can grow in the holding tank, especially in warm climates. Ultraviolet is sometimes added to ensure bacterial and viral sterilization. RO units are usually supplemented with both before and after charcoal filters.

Disadvantages. RO units save a bundle on electricity, but they use a lot of water, about 4-6 gallons for every 1 gallon cleaned. Most membranes need to be changed in one to three years. As the membrane ages, its capacity to clean decreases. Contaminants that would be removed by a new RO, may not be removed by an old one. Without a water test, there is no way to know for sure. The lifetime and performance of the semipermeable membrane depends on the amount of use, water pressure, temperature, pH (alkalinity), sediment, and mineral content. These variables, plus its slow drop-by-drop operation and high water usage are the challenges of this technology for household treatment.

Unit prices range between $400 and $1500. Replacement membranes cost $100 or more. Supplemental carbon filters cost $30–$70 and usually have a 6 month life.

Home Distillation Systems

Distillation is the process of boiling water into steam and then collecting the steam back into water. Of all the water treatment methods, distillation is the most independent, requiring the least amount of supplementation from other methods and covering the broadest range of contaminants. It is the crown jewel of water purification. Even though carbon filters and reverse osmosis units far outsell them, as stand alone devices, distillers make the purest water. In fact, it is the only kind of water laboratory scientists use because they must make sure their water has nothing in it that will influence their experiments.

Distillation Effectively Removes:

- All bacteria and microorganisms including viruses
- Soluble inorganic salts such as fluoride, sodium, nitrates
- Organic chemicals like pesticides, PCBs, THMs
- Radionuclides
- Heavy metals such as lead, mercury, arsenic, cadmium, etc.
- Soluble minerals: calcium, phosphorous, magnesium, etc.

It has been said that distillation is the most natural of all water purification methods. Rainwater is nature's distillation method. Water on the ground evaporates and rises into the air as vapor (steam) until it reaches a certain altitude where it cools and falls

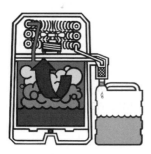

The process of distillation mimics the natural process of evaporation and condensation that ultimately creates rain. In an unpolluted world, rain is distilled water.

back to earth as rain. Unfortunately, our air quality is not as pure as in the days of the Garden of Eden. So today, our rain passes through a lot of dirty air on its way down including such contaminants as sulfuric acid and nitric acid which make the infamous acid rain.

Distillers work the same way, but without the air pollution. First the water is boiled, then cooled and condensed back into water. The boiling is usually done in a pot-like stainless steel chamber. Most distillers use electricity to heat the water, although you can find some that boil on top of a gas stove and even others that use solar heat. The boiled off steam is then captured and passed through a condensing chamber. This is usually a coiled tube typically made of stainless steel, glass or aluminum. Some distillers surround the tube with cool water that lowers the temperature of the steam thereby creating water droplets. Most distillers, however, use fans rather than water to cool down the steam. The water vapor is then collected drop by drop into a sterile container. This natural process takes time, between 2 and 4 hours to collect one gallon!

Advantages of Distillers

Distillers effectively remove bacteria, viruses, mineral salts such as fluoride, sodium, nitrates, asbestos, and all minerals including heavy metals. The water has no odor, no color, and no taste. This is the nature of distilled water. Prices for home distillers range from $300 to $1,500, so there are differences that involve the features of the appliance and the quality of the water.

What to Consider When Shopping for A Home Distiller

- Price
- Size
- Rate (speed) of distillation
- Water or air cooled
- Quantity of water used
- Amount of electricity used
- Self-cleaning or manual

- Automatic or manual input
- Hot & cold water dispenser
- Built-in collection container
- Safety of materials used
- Elimination of toxic gases
- Pre & post charcoal filters

Features of Different Distillers

There is a great diversity of distillers in the marketplace. This is most likely because there are many different ways to condense water. It is so simple, you can even make your own distiller with a basic chemistry set. Since the 1960s when water pollution scares made front page headlines, clean water companies have poured into the market. Diversity is typically a wonderful asset, but when shopping for a distiller, it can also mean confusion.

The first thing most people consider when shopping for a distiller is price. The price of a distiller has much to do with the volume of water it can produce and how fast it can produce it. Beyond that, price is very dependent on extra features such as cold and hot water dispensers, ice cube makers, automatic on and off, size of reservoir, stainless steel vs. aluminum or plastic components, etc. Buy only the features you need and you will save money. A little ingenuity will also help. Stainless steel, for example, is expensive and a stainless steel collection reservoir can cost from $50 to $500. But a 5 gallon polycarbonate bottle—the kind you find in office water dispensers—costs less than $20. Large glass bottles are another economical alternative.

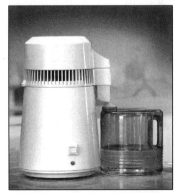

An affordable countertop distiller that is filled by hand and does not require any plumbing.

Cleaning

Some other features are more essential. Self-cleaning or easy cleaning is very important. Because distillers remove minerals and heavy metals, they can build up scale in their boiling chambers, especially if you have hard water. It is common to be lazy about cleaning out the scale, but also unwise to continue to distill from an excessively scaley chamber that might affect the purity of the output. Scale solvents are a good way to clean your distiller and are easy to use. They are readily available at housewares stores (for irons and humidifiers) or from your distiller dealer. It is also nice to have a boiling chamber with easy access so you can go in there and scrub if you need to. Some distillers have self-cleaning mechanisms that constantly flush out the dirty water, thereby stretching the time between cleanings to as few as once per year.

Water, Air, and Electricity

A few distillers are water cooled, most are air cooled, and some have both. If a distiller is water cooled, you will use approximately 6 gallons of coolant water to make 1 gallon of the pure water. This may not be ideal if water is scarce or expensive. Air cooling is done by fans and in some models, wastes no water at all. However, fans do add some "white" noise and slightly increase the use of electricity.

Speaking of electricity, distillers typically use between 500 and 1500 watts per hour. Some use as much as 3000 watts, others use none at all; they use gas. To get the model with the lowest wattage, however, is not necessarily best. There is a ratio between the use of electricity and rate of distillation that is important to balance. Low wattage machines, 500 watts for example, may take 6 hours to make one gallon. That adds up to 3500 watts per gallon. On the other hand, a 1500 watt machine, makes a gallon in 2 hours for a total of 3000 watts per gallon. This relationship between electricity and rate of distillation determines your machine's efficiency and economy. The average distilling time of an efficient, high volume distiller is between 2 and 3 hours per gallon and approximately 3 kilowatt-hours per gallon. Your final cost should be approximately 25 cents per gallon including the cost of replacing the accompanying charcoal filters.

Automatic Operation

Automatic feeding is a valuable feature. Some distillers connect to your cold water line or faucet and receive their water from it. The distiller adjusts the incoming flow of water automatically through a valve. Better machines also have the ability to shut off if, for some reason, the house water supply fails. Automatic feeding is far more convenient than the "pot boiler" type of distiller that needs to be filled manually every gallon or so. However, it is again a question of need. A small household of two persons may do very well with a manual feed machine. It is a question of budget, lifestyle, and usage.

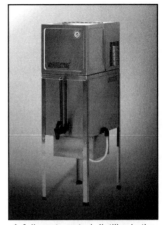

A fully automated distiller is the epitome of convenience. These machines are just as valuable as other large appliances that serve the home and in fact, can join them in the utility room.

Importance of Quality Materials

The materials used in the distiller you choose should, of course, be nontoxic. Aluminum or low grade plastics may break down and contaminate your distilled water. Plastic exteriors, or plastic and aluminum boiling chambers may be perfectly acceptable because in the end, the distilled water never touches them. While stainless steel and glass are the finest materials, having them in every part of a machine is very expensive. Shop for a distiller that uses them only where you need it. Plastic tubing is common in distillers, and is safe. Such plastic is made of high quality, surgical grade material that can withstand temperatures of up to 600 degrees! These days, plastics are so diversified, we must learn to distinguish between those that are harmful and helpful.

Elimination of Gases

From the standpoint of health, the most important function of a distiller is its ability to eliminate various gases and volatile organic compounds. These are liquids that have boiling points lower or approximately the same as water and can thus be carried over with the purified water. Chloroform is one example of a pollutant that can be transported over with the distilled water. This is the Achilles' heel of distillation. But quality distillation systems have different ways of dealing with it.

Carbon filters can assist the distiller in eliminating these gases. Carbon excels in adsorbing gases and volatile organic compounds. The combination of the two methods makes a perfect marriage in water purification. The carbon takes care of the gases and the distiller virtually eliminates heavy metals and inorganic compounds. The boiling process of distillation also kills the bacteria that would ordinarily breed in a charcoal filter. In effect, each method fills in for the other's weaknesses.

Filters can be located on the distiller in either of two places. In an auto-fill distiller, a prefilter is situated on the line between the faucet and the unit or under the sink on the cold water line. A post carbon filter is located on the distilled water exit just before the collecting bottle. The post filter, however, is subject to some of the same problems of all simple carbon filters. They can breed bacteria. On the positive side, the likelihood of breeding bacteria is limited since the source water has already been sterilized (boiled) and the slow drop by drop action through the carbon affords the water maximum contact time and therefore greatest adsorption. Post filters are inexpensive and are included with many distillers, although you can run the machine with or without it. Prefilters are more sophisticated and more expensive. Even if your distiller does not come with a prefilter, you can still add it as an independent unit.

The most common method for eliminating gases in distillers is the pre-boiling chamber and escape vent. The water to be distilled is first detained in a boiling chamber for several minutes (the length of time depends on the design). The longer it boils, the more toxic gases escape through the vent. Even here, there are differences between good distillers and bad. Poorly designed distillers allow for very short detention periods. Others do not provide a sufficient enough venting area.

Disadvantages of Distillers

Although distillation is the most thorough method of water purification, like all other methods, it has its disadvantages. Probably the biggest complaint about distillers is the inconvenience of not having water on demand. From the point of view of the average American surrounded by appliances designed to make their kitchen life more convenient, the requirement of plugging something in and waiting hours to get a gallon, is a bit much. High output distillers take an average of 3 hours to make a gallon of water. Countertop distillers can take as long as 6 hours to make a gallon. Of course, if you buy a fully automatic distiller, you will never have to wait for your water.

As mentioned in our discussion on electricity, most distillers are electric. They will have an impact on your electric bill according to the efficiency of the machine. Before you purchase a distiller, find out the cost per gallon to operate it. Some machines are definitely more economical than others. In some areas, running your distiller overnight may take advantage of lower utility rates. Summertime can be an uncomfortable time to run a distiller, depending on its location. Electric rates are often higher and heat and humidity from the distiller only add to the battle between your air conditioner and your sweat glands. On the other hand, most appliances in your house use electricity. Your air conditioner, dryer, and refrigerator all use lots of electricity, but you would

---

Disadvantages of Distillers

- Takes hours to make water
- Often uses electricity
- Can create heat & humidity
- More of an investment than a simple carbon filter
- Requires water storage
- Generally bigger than carbon filters
- Possibly less convenient
- May have a different taste

---

never eliminate them because they are essential. Pure water is also essential and certainly worth paying for. And the cost of producing it at home is less than buying it.

Water is another form of energy that distillers use. On the average, water cooled distillers use 6 gallons of waste water in the process of making one gallon of distilled water. If water is scarce or expensive in your area, it may not be practical to own this kind of distiller. A fan cooled distiller saves water by cooling with air.

Of course, you must consider size and price when shopping for a distiller. There are countertop models for $300; and there are completely automated floor models that cost in the $1,500 range and need to be located in your laundry room, basement, or garage.

Probably the last straw for thirsty Americans is the typical complaint about its "lack of taste." Real pure water has no taste. However, even a neutral taste tastes like something, relative to everything else. Of course, if you buy it in a flaccid HDPE plastic bottle (#2 in the triangle on the bottom), it will have a taste—a taste of plastic! Distilled water leaves no aftertaste because it is free of the chemicals and impurities that create taste. Most people quickly get used to this "non-taste;" many actually prefer it, and others don't even notice it. Taste is a subjective experience. After drinking your favorite water consistently, every other water tends to taste odd.

Storage of Distilled Water

One more disadvantage of distillers is not in the making of the water, but in the storage of it. Distilled water, like any food, is subject to spoilage if left open and unrefrigerated for many days. Storage bottles should be sterilized so that bacteria cannot build up in them. This can be as simple as rinsing with hot water, if it is a half or one gallon jar. A five gallon tank, however, requires more work. Large tanks or five gallon jugs can be sterilized with a small amount of chlorine bleach. Add one tablespoon to one gallon of water and let stand for one hour. Rinse thoroughly afterwards. As an alternative to chlorine, you can use hydrogen peroxide or boiling water. For long term storage, keep your water refrigerated. If using a five gallon reservoir, use up your water within a week and sterilize the reservoir periodically.

While cleaning these large bottles can be a nuisance, extracting the water from them is yet another problem. Special pumps and dispenser stands are available for 5 gallon bottles. Again, this raises the issue of proper sterilization as well as floor space. It is inconveniences like these that prompt the plea, "Wouldn't it be nice to just press a lever and get a drink of water?"

Convenient Distilled Water

Top of the line distillers provide all the conveniences you need, but they are bigger. These units are well suited for a utility room, basement, or garage. Fully automated machines turn on when their reservoirs are low and turn off when they are full. Water is piped from the distiller to the kitchen and/or bathroom wherever drinking water is required. In the kitchen, there is a water fountain spigot that delivers water. These distillers are so sophisticated, they can even deliver ice—gourmet ice! These models serve large families and are the epitome of convenience. Yes, they are the most expensive machines and involve the most complex installation. But if Americans put a fraction of the investment into their water that they now spend on their cars or furnishings in their homes, we'd all be a lot healthier for it.

Distilled Water vs. Spring Water

One of the greatest controversies in the arena of water and health has to do with the desirability of drinking spring water vs. distilled water. Spring water has a natural mineral content. Distilled water has no minerals and because it is sterile, it is often referred to as "lifeless" water. The spring water advocates say spring water provides necessary minerals. They also say because distilled water is void of minerals, it robs them from the body. The distilled water advocates say food is a better source of organic minerals than water and the inorganic minerals in water are not fully utilized by the body. Like most controversies, there is truth on both sides. However, a clearer understanding can be found by putting these truths in perspective.

Distilled water has been described by its adversaries as dead water because it is sterile, with no mineral or organic life in it. For this reason it is highly unstable and will attract any organic material that comes in contact with it. Once it is "contaminated" by organic matter, it becomes stable. This is the property that gives distilled water its alleged ability to leach minerals from the body. However, distilled water cannot attract organically bound minerals from our bones and cells. Minerals found in spring water are inorganic; they are run off from stone, soil, and rock dissolved in water. Scientists tell us that only plants can convert inorganic minerals to a useable form which can be absorbed by our digestive tract. Fresh fruits and vegetables are our best source of absorbable minerals. Distilled water can "leach" inorganic minerals, but as soon as it comes in contact with the contents of our stomach, it is immediately neutralized. Thus, although it is technically correct to claim that distilled water can leach, it has no practical impact on human health. Tens of thousands of kidney patients using distilled water in their dialysis machines attest to the fact that distilled water will not leach organic minerals from our bodies.

The Leaching Controversy

Here are some further points to help interpret the truths on both sides of this controversy. First of all, never buy distilled water in HDPE flexible plastic containers (#2 on the bottom of the bottle). Because of its unstable nature, distilled water will pick up plastic from the walls of this container and it will be noticeable in the taste. On the other hand, you can take advantage of distilled water's naturally aggressive, chelating ability and put something nourishing in it. A few grains of rice per gallon of water, for example, will stabilize the distilled water in minutes and add organic minerals to it. You will have produced, in effect, your own homemade mineral water. Now it is "alive" with nutrients and organic minerals and should be refrigerated or drunk within a few days. It is, in fact, more dependable than spring or mineral water, because you can trust that it comes from an absolutely pure source. Compare that to all the unknowns of choosing between the various brands of bottled waters.

You can no more digest inorganic minerals
than you can dirt.—Paul Bragg, N.D., Ph.D.[49]

This principle of stabilization also applies to any kitchen use of distilled water. Any time you use distilled water as an ingredient of a dressing or a soup, it is immediately stabilized. When you drink distilled water, it will likewise stabilize as it mixes with the contents of your stomach. Only when you drink distilled water repeatedly on a fast can it have the potential to leach minerals from the body, and then only when the process of genuine starvation has commenced. This extreme circumstance affirms the mineral-leaching theory, but it bears no relevance to normal human nutrition.

Here are some questions to consider: how much and what does distilled water leach out? Does it take out more minerals than what comes in? Lastly, are there any advantages to this leaching?

As it turns out, one glass of fresh carrot juice contains more biologically available minerals—in the organic assimilable form—than gallons of the finest spring water. Not only that, but minerals are in a constant state of flux within our bodies. We eliminate volumes of minerals every day and volumes more come in. Minerals are "pulled out" from foods that are much more aggressive than distilled water—vinegar, vitamin C, acid fruits, herbs, and diuretics like coffee and soft drinks. Even if it was possible for distilled water to go into our bones and pull out calcium, there would be plenty more coming along from our diet to replace it . If you are concerned about minerals, make your own "homemade" mineral water from distilled water. Or better yet, eat whole foods and drink plenty of fresh fruit and vegetable juices. And don't forget your sea vegetables—kelp, dulse, nori, hijiki, etc. They are our best dietary source of organic minerals.

How Can We Keep our Water Pure?

Pure water is, next to oxygen, the most fundamental element necessary for life. Its availability is an inalienable right that does not have to be written in the Constitution. The contamination of our water supply by government and industry threatens the ecology of our planet and the health of all living things. If you want to do something about it, clean up your own drinking water first. Then, consider joining the fight by supporting your favorite environmental preservationist organization such as *Greenpeace, Sierra Club, Audubon Society, Environmental Defense Fund, etc.* Their job, and yours, is to remind your legislators and fellow citizens about this precious treasure—our natural waters—and to protect forevermore. Legislators are overwhelmed by the persuasions of government and industry, but they need to hear your voice, too. The environmental organizations will help you get your message across. You need them and they need you. Together, we can stop this illfated pollution and rescue our planet's greatest resource.

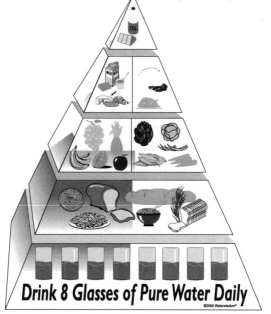

Drink 8 Glasses of Pure Water Daily

Footnotes

1. *For Lifelong Gains, Just Add Water. Repeat.* Brody, Jane E. New York Times, July 11, 2000.

2. Report from Nutrition Information Center at the *New York Hospital-Cornell Medical Center,* May 11, 1998.

3. Cornell University Medical Center, Nutrition Information Center. Survey conducted by Yankelovich Partners. Underwritten by The International Bottled Water Association (IBWA). Reported in *Alternative Medicine Magazine.* June 3, 2000

4. National Soft Drink Assoc. web site, www.NSDA.org.

5. *American Journal Clinical Nutrition.* 1995;62(suppl):178S-94S.

6. Hiller WD, et al. Medical and physiological considerations in triathlons. *Am J Sports Med* 1987 Mar;(2):164-7.

7. Wenk C, et al. Methodological studies of the estimation of loss of sodium, potassium, calcium and magnesium through the skin during a 10 km run. *Z Ernahrungswiss* 1993 Dec;(4):301-7.

8. Tarnopolsky MA, et al. Mixed carbohydrate supplementation increases carbohydrate oxidation and endurance exercise performance and attenuates potassium accumulation. *Int J Sport Nutr* 1996 Dec;(4):323-36.

9. *Your Body's Many Cries for Water* by Fereydoon Batmanghelidj, MD Global Health Solutions, Falls Church, VA. 800-759-3999. www.WaterCure.com

10. *ABC of Asthma, Allergies and Lupus* by Dr. Fereydoon Batmanghelidj, MD Global Health Solutions, Falls Church, VA. 800-759-3999. www.WaterCure.com

11. *ABC of Asthma, Allergies and Lupus* by Dr. Fereydoon Batmanghelidj, MD. pgs. 142-145. Global Health Solutions, Falls Church, VA. 800-759-3999.

12. Ann Louise Gittleman, M.S., C.N.S. *Healthy Talk Newsletter.* December, 1996, p.5. and *Guess What Came to Dinner : Parasites and Your Health*, ppbk, 194pgs. 1993. Avery Pub Group.

13. *ABC of Asthma, Allergies and Lupus* by Dr. Fereydoon Batmanghelidj, MD. pgs. 38-43. Global Health Solutions, Falls Church, VA. 800-759-3999.

14. Morris, RD *"Drinking Water and Cancer"* Environmental Health Perspectives 1995. 103 Suppl 8: 225-231.

15. Kleiners, SM "Water: An essential but overlooked nutrient" *Journal of the American Dietetic Association.* 1999. 99:200-206.

16. Hydrotherapy. *Nutrition Science News,* May, 1999. Boulder, CO.

17. Chaitow, L. *The Body/Mind Purification Program.* New York: Simon and Schuster, 1990.

18. *Water Technology Magazine,* April 14, 1999.

19. "Tracking Ground Water's Unwelcome Guests" by Robert A. Soar. *New York Times.* 11/23/99.

20. *Dateline NBC. 1994. Sept. 20, 27, 28.* Journal of the American Chiropractic Association. March 2000. Pg 23.

21. "Wetter is Better," *Better Nutrition Magazine,* Aug, 1998, pg. 37-38. Sabot Publishing, Stamford, CT.

22. *American Academy of Anti-Aging Medicine* is a non-profit medical society dedicated solely to the advancement of longevity related medicine. 773-528-4333, fax 773-528-1043. http://www.worldhealth.net

23. National Health Alert, *Stream of Success Magazine,* April, 2000. p. 5. Published by Multi-Pure, Las Vegas, NV.

24. *Journal of Dental Research* 1968. 47:407.

25. *The New Drug Story,* by Morris A. Bealle, Columbia Publishing Company, 1958. Pg 144.

26. *Fluoridation: The Great Dilemma,* by George L. Waldbott, M.D., Coronado Press, Inc., Kansas, 1978

27. *Fluoride.* 23(2):55-67. 1990.

28. *Community Dentistry and Oral Epidemiology.* 13:37-41. 1985. *Community Health Studies.* 11:85-89. 1987.

29. *Mutation Research.* 223:181-205. 1989.

30. *IRCS Medical Science Library Compendium.* 9(11):1021-1122. 1981.

31. *Archives of Internal Medicine.* 75:745-747. 1971.

32. *Lifesavers Guide To Fluoridation,* by John Yiamouyiannis, Ph.D Published by The National Health Federation, Box 688, Monrovia, CA 91016. 213-357-2181.

33. *Journal of the American Chemical Society.* 103:24-28. 1981.

34. *Environmental & Molecular Mutagenisis.* 21:309-318. 1993.

35. *New England Journal of Medicine,* March 22, 1990. *Fluoride,* 6:4-18. 1973.

36. Gareth W. Dodd. Chemicals, pharmaceuticals found below wastewater plants. *U.S. Water News,* Vol. 17, No. 6, page 1, 12.

37. Ibid.

38. "Tough to Swallow, How Pesticide Companies Profit from Poisoning America's Tap Water," *The Environmental Working Group Report,* 8/12/97.

39. *Acid Procrastination,* Editorial, The New York Times, September 2, 1984

40. Grenawitzke, H. "Controlling Contamination in Drinking Water Treatment Chemicals." *Waterworks,* 2(1):1-5. March, 1998.

41. Ibid.

42. "It's Only Water, Right?" *Consumer Reports Magazine,* 8/2000. Pg.16-20. "The Selling of H₂0" *Consumer Reports Magazine,* September, 1980

43. "Drinking Water," Editor John Lobell, *Natural Living Newsletter,* No. 19. New York, NY.

44. "Water Filters" *Consumer Reports Magazine,* February, 1983

45. . A comparison of the Bactericidal Activity of Ozone and Chlorine against E. Coli at 1 degree Fahrenheit. by R.H. Fetner, and R.S. Ingols. J. *Gen. Microbial,* 1956, vol. 15, p.381.

46. . Some Chemical Viewpoints on the Ozonation of Water, by W. Stumm, *Schweiz, Zeitsch. Hydrol,* 1956, vol. 18 No. 2, p.201.

47. . Disinfection and Sterilization of Sewage by Ozone, by S. Miller, et al., *Advances in Chemistry Series,* 1959, vol. 21 p.381.

48. . Ozone Treatment of Secondary Effluents from Wastewater Treatment Plants, by D. Huibers, et al. Report No. TWRC-4, *Advanced Waste Treatment Reservoir Laboratory* and the Air Reduction Company. 4/1969.

49. . Paul Bragg, N.D., Ph.D., Water : The Shocking Truth That Can Save Your Life. Ppbk. 1999. *Health Science.*

Resources

Other Books About Water

Your Body's Many Cries for Water, by F. Batmanghelidj, MD. Global Health Solutions, Falls Church, VA. 800-759-3999. www.WaterCure.com The definitive text on the health benefits of proper hydration.

ABC of Asthma, Allergies and Lupus, by F. Batmanghelidj, MD. Global Health Solutions, Falls Church, VA. 800-759-3999. www.WaterCure.com

Water: The Shocking Truth That Can Save Your Life, by Paul Bragg, N.D., Ph.D., Ppbk. 1999. Health Science.

Water Conditioning & Purification Magazine. A comprehensive trade publication serving all facets of the water industry. http://www.wcp.net

EPA's Safe Drinking Water Hotline, 800-426-4791 or visit their website at www.EPA.gov/safewater

Pollution Prevention Information Clearinghouse (PPIC). An information resource on pollution issues from the Environmental Protection Agency (EPA) 202-260-1023.

Home Testing Labs

National Testing Labs. Cleveland, OH. 800-458-3330. www.WaterCheck.com Home water testing.

Spectrum Labs, Inc. St. Paul, MN. 800-447-5221. www.Spectrum-labs.com Home water testing.

Suburban Water Testing. Temple, PA 800-433-6595. www.H20test.com Home water testing.

Watertest Corporation. Manchester, NH 800-426-8378. www.WaterCheck.com Home water testing.

Water Quality Association. This international association (with members in over 70 countries) is a resource for standards in the water treatment industry and a valuable source for worldwide networking opportunities. http://www.wqa.org

Bottled Water Web™ This is a web portal for the bottled water industry where you will find extensive information about bottled water including both trade and consumers news and articles. http://www.bottledwaterweb.com

American Academy of Anti-Aging Medicine is a non-profit medical society dedicated to the advancement of longevity related medicine. Its membership includes physicians and scientists from around the world. Membership is open to the public. 773-528-4333, fax 528-1043. http://www.worldhealth.net

Index

Other Books

By Steve Meyerowitz

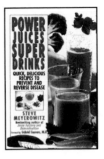

Power Juices Super Drinks
Quick, Delicious Recipes to Reverse and
Prevent Disease. March, 2000.

Wheatgrass Nature's Finest Medicine
*The Complete Guide to Using Grass Foods
& Juices to Revitalize Your Health.* 1999.

Juice Fasting & Detoxification
*Use the Healing Power of Fresh Juice to Feel Young and Look
Great* 1999.

Food Combining and Digestion
*A Rational Approach to Combining What You Eat to Maximize
Digestion and Health* 1996.

Sproutman's Kitchen Garden Cookbook
*Sprout Breads, Cookies, Soups, Salads & 250 other Low Fat,
Dairy Free Vegetarian Recipes* 1999.

Sprouts the Miracle Food
The Complete Guide to Sprouting 1999.

Sproutman's "Turn the Dial" Sprout Chart
A Field Guide to Growing and Eating Sprouts 1998.

Clinician's Complete Reference to Complementary/Alternative Medicine.
Steve Meyerowitz, co-author. Edited by Donald W. Novey,
M.D. 2000.

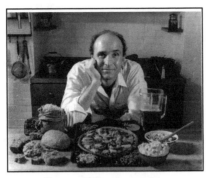

Steve Meyerowitz

Steve Meyerowitz began his journey to better health in 1975 to correct a lifelong chronic condition of severe allergies and asthma. After two months of eating a raw foods–vegetarian diet, his symptoms disappeared. Steve endured 20 years of disappointment with conventional medicine before he restored his health through his own program of purification, lifestyle adjustment, exercise, fasting, juicing and living foods.

Over the years, he has lived on and experimented with many so called 'extreme' diet/lifestyles including raw foods, fruitarianism, sprouts, dairy and flourless vegetarianism and fasting. In 1977, he was pronounced "Sproutman" by *Vegetarian Times Magazine* in a feature article that explored his innovative sprouting ideas and recipes.

After 10 years as a music and comedy entertainer, he made a complete lifestyle change for his health. In 1980, he opened *The Sprout House*, a "no-cooking school" in New York City. There, he began a formal program of teaching kitchen gardening and the preparation of gourmet sprouted and vegetarian foods. Steve has invented two home sprouters, the *Flax Sprout Bag* and the *Kitchen Garden Salad Grower*. He founded the Sprout House, a company supplying home growing kits and organic sprouting seeds.

Steve has been featured on the *QVC, Home Shopping Network, TV Food Network,* in *Prevention, Organic Gardening* and *Flower & Garden Magazines.* He and his family, including three little sprouts, live in the Berkshire mountains of Mass.